I0510261

The Nurse Leader

Leadership in Healthcare Organizations

The Ultimate Guide to Become the Boss who
Everyone Wants

Grey Daniel

© Copyright 2019 by Grey Daniel
All rights reserved.

This document is geared towards providing exact and reliable information with regards to the topic and issue covered. The publication is sold with the idea that the publisher is not required to render accounting, officially permitted, or otherwise, qualified services. If advice is necessary, legal or professional, a practiced individual in the profession should be ordered.

- From a Declaration of Principles which was accepted and approved equally by a Committee of the American Bar Association and a Committee of Publishers and Associations.

In no way is it legal to reproduce, duplicate, or transmit any part of this document in either electronic means or in printed format. Recording of this publication is strictly prohibited and any storage of this document is not allowed unless with written permission from the publisher. All rights reserved.

The information provided herein is stated to be truthful and consistent, in that any liability, in terms of inattention or otherwise, by any usage or abuse of any policies, processes, or directions contained within is the solitary and utter responsibility of the recipient reader. Under no circumstances will any legal responsibility or blame be held against the publisher for any reparation, damages, or monetary loss due to the information herein, either directly or indirectly.

Respective authors own all copyrights not held by the publisher.

The information herein is offered for informational purposes solely, and is universal as so. The presentation of the information is without contract or any type of guarantee assurance.

The trademarks that are used are without any consent, and the publication of the trademark is without permission or backing by the trademark owner. All trademarks and brands within this book are for clarifying purposes only and are the owned by the owners themselves, not affiliated with this document.

Disclaimer

All erudition contained in this book is given for informational and educational purposes only. The author is not in any way accountable for any results or outcomes that emanate from using this material. Constructive attempts have been made to provide information that is both accurate and effective, but the author is not bound for the accuracy or use/misuse of this information.

Table of contents

INTRODUCTION

On the off chance that they're on day shift they touch base at the clinic or office around 6:00 am to be prepared to set up a case at 7:00 am. This gives them an opportunity to change into scrubs and read their calendar. The calendar is their fate for the following 8-12 hours. They take a look at the huge board by the front work area to see whether they're the scrub nurse that day, or the orderly.

The primary reason they're searching the board for is to see which specialist they'll be working with. This straightforward thing can represent the moment of truth in their day. There are both great and awful specialists, much the same as some other cut of the populace. "Please God, don't let it be so and so."

Specialists can be benevolent, yet their abilities might be repulsive. Or, on the other hand, they can be incredible surgeons, however genuine monsters. Ideally that day you will be working with every one of the specialists who are both cordial and great at what they do... be that as it may, it isn't likely.

If you're appointed to be the orderly, at that point you snatch your scrub tech/nurse, and you both go to find your first case truck of the day. This could be anyplace in the chaos of different trucks that have been loaded up with things required for different cases. Well, what a delight! This is the point where you have a major ortho case and half of the instruments aren't sterile and should be flashed. Better yet, half of the things on the tendency sheet are absent.

You need to run and find them while your scrub nurse is opening the clean field. When you return you "hit the dance floor with your scrub nurse." Not really, however to "hit the dance floor with your scrub nurse" really implies you help the scrub nurse tie her/his clean outfit. They can't do this all alone, or it would render them unsterile, for coming to despite their good faith.

You at that point must check everything, including every one of the instruments, raytec, laps, needles, and edges. Keep in mind this is done between 6:30 am and 7:00 am. Heaven forbid you lose a lap or any of the above things. It's a nightmare when you lose anything. I've been in situations where we were removing a lap wipe, a needle or an instrument; these cases are so much fun.

During situations where the specialist has recently left a wipe inside the patient, you unquestionably need a touch of wintergreen on your veil, or you are probably going to vomit your guts up! (What's more, that is putting it mildly).

Anyway, once everything is checked, your scrub nurse is upbeat, your OR bed is sheeted and all the hardware is in the room, it's a great opportunity to go out and welcome the patient.

CHAPTER ONE

Effective communication

All that we do has something to do with correspondence. Much of the time we think it is something that happens when we are talking or listening. We recognize that the individual hearing the information doesn't generally have to be accessible (for instance seeing the TV or listening to the radio) anyway we understand that for correspondence to have happened, something probably happened inside the group of spectators. It moreover has to do with understanding the desire for the individual talking and affirmation of that information or the significance proposed by the speaker.

Let say it offers differences and sets up regular timeframes to put these out and address them. In the two connections and groups, a setting can be set inside where differences can normally be examined. Whenever this is done in an exploratory manner, it turns into a chance to share alternate points of view and explain errors. If we just wait until these differences in one way or another meddle with accomplishing a result, then the discussion turns into a troublesome one where much is on the line, feelings vary and emotions are high.

Setting aside a few minutes to talk about differences when everyone is not pressed to get a result immediately, enables trust to be established in a relationship. At the point when critical discussions happen later on, there is money in the bank, enabling differences to be investigated without fighting. When enlisting representatives, consideration is centered around what they can or may have the option to do. Extraordinary lengths are taken to relate existing capacities and aptitudes against proportions of future execution. Character and group job types are additionally used to assess the probability of an individual meeting the activity prerequisites and functioning well inside the group.

However, social standards regularly only become obvious 'at work'. If a group culture is created which empowers the exchange of the implications behind communicated and certain qualities and standards, then the opportunity exists for advancement and imaginative methods for taking care of the issues. The same is true when enlisting a helper - turning into a silent communicator enables differences to be analyzed without danger, scorn or opposition.

Anyone who has ever been in love encounters a culture of two, every individual tuned to one another's dog whistle that only the other individual can hear. Too bad, if the relationship finishes in tears, those common implications some way or another don't appear to matter. In any case, what was accomplished in the relationship was an encounter of seen 'we-ness'. The probability of the relationship going on and being supported after some time, has a great deal to do with the capacity of the partners to endure differences that beforehand were not evident in the special first night meeting.

Despite everything they may find their hearts moved by a common tune or commonly delighted in film, yet for a sound relationship to build up, each must understand their various characters. Moreover in relationships, the cohesiveness of a group relies upon the degree to which the individuals maintain standards that are imperative to them as a group. Generational contrasts make group working testing when individuals from various ages are attempting to agree on how best to cooperate. These various desires for work and life sway colossally on cutting edge hierarchical conduct and together with high turnover and the reality of progress and different vocations over a lifetime, sway on the network which we call work.

In any case, for all groups to work viably a feeling of 'we' must rise up which requires an authoritative style that empowers shared implications that produce gainful outcomes and individual and group fulfillment.

Everything is Communication

All that we do has something to do with correspondence. Much of the time we think it is something that happens when we are talking or tuning in. We recognize that the individual hearing the information doesn't generally ought to be accessible (for instance seeing the TV or tuning in on the radio) anyway we understand that for correspondence to have happened, something probably happened inside the group of spectators. It moreover has to do with understanding the desire for the individual talking and affirmation of that information or the significance proposed by the speaker.

Let say it offer contrasts and set up standard occasions to convey and address In the two connections and groups, a setting can be set inside which contrasts can normally be examined. Whenever done in an exploratory manner, it turns into a chance to share alternate points of view and explain errors. On the off chance that we just hold up until contrasts some way or another meddle with accomplishing a result, at that point the discussion turns into a troublesome one where a lot is on the line, feelings vary and feelings are raised. Setting aside a few minutes to talk about contrasts when each are not squeezed to get a result immediately, enables trust to create in a relationship. At that point when critical discussions happen later on, there is credit in the bank, enabling contrasts to be investigated without strife. When enrolling representatives, consideration is centered around what can or may have the option to do. Extraordinary lengths are taken to relate existing capacities and aptitudes against proportions of future execution. Character and group job types are additionally used to assess the probability of an individual gathering the activity prerequisites and functioning admirably inside the group. Be that as it may, social and social standards regularly just become obvious 'at work'. On the off chance that a group culture is created which empower exchange of the implications behind communicated and certain qualities and standards, at that point opportunity exist for advancement and imaginative methods for taking care of issues. The equivalent is genuine when enrolling an accomplice - turning into a quiet communicator enables contrasts to be analyzed without danger, scorn or opposition.

Anyone who has ever been infatuated encounters a culture of two, every individual tuned to one another's pooch whistle that solitary the other individual can hear. Too bad, if the relationship finishes in tears, those common implications some way or another don't appear to correspond. In any case, what was made in the association was an encounter of seen 'we-ness'. The probability of the relationship proceeding and being supported after some time, has a great deal to do with the capacity of the accomplices to endure contrasts that beforehand were not evident in the special first night organize. Despite everything they may discover their hearts moved by a common tune or commonly delighted in film, yet for a sound relationship to build up, each must understand their various characters. Moreover in associations, the cohesiveness of a group relies upon the degree to which the individuals maintain standards that are imperative to them as a gathering. Generational contrasts make group working testing when individuals from various ages are attempting to concur on how best to cooperate. These various desires for work and life sway colossally on cutting edge hierarchical conduct and together with high turnover and the truth of progress and different vocations over a lifetime, sway on the network which we call work. In any case, for all groups to work viably there must build up a feeling of 'we' which requires an authority style that empowered shared implications that produce gainful outcomes and individual and aggregate fulfillment.

What Is Communication?

Communication is the cash with which we explore our own and expert connections. The difference between good and bad communicators does not depend on aptitudes capacity alone. At the point when an individual has a decent association with themself and assumes full liability as far as it concerns them in making their external reality, they are ready to change and improve their realationships.

By creating a self-doubting mentality that continually asks, 'What is my part in creating what's going on here?' they are ready to change something important to themself as opposed to seek after conditions to change or reprimand others for their encounters. The reason that an abnormal state of mindfulness is fundamental in powerful communication is that there are hidden, oblivious components that impact our behavior to such an extent (if not more) than known ones.

This is clear when an individual understands they continue drawing in comparable results throughout their life and where comparable games, movies and elements continue happening in their life which they feel too weak to change. Without changing one's interior discourse, testing the inward saboteur and finding the source of one's damaging, self-disrupting gehavior, an individual is destined to get comparable results - paying little mind to whether those results help them in getting the outcomes they need.

Listening to a powerful communicator is only conceivable when aptitudes preparations are joined with an individual creating an on-going capacity to act naturally intelligent, assume liability and in each discussion, see their part in creating the outcomes they get. When these capacities are consolidated, they legitimately add to an individual accomplishing the connections they need, as well as making them incredible communicators who have effect and impact on others.

Via communication, individuals trade. Communication is a basic trait of human life, which is the reason we as a whole invest a large portion of our energy either getting or asking for information. Absence of communication causes strains and decimates individual and nursing relationships. The capacity to trade information or have a discussion with others is pivotal to the achievement of the individual, family or nursing organization. It ought to be noted, notwithstanding, that it is one thing to try to communicate, yet entirely something else to convey viably.

Ineffectual communication for the most part brings about disappointment, as it doesn't evoke the ideal reaction in the type of input from the recipient. This is the most despicable aspect of many nursing organizations. Many supervisors do try to communicate, however regularly they are not success. Absence of the ability to Communication adequately with respect to bosses is the reason behind the disappointment of many organizations. Each firm or nursing organization needs a successful Communication arrangement to work appropriately and accomplish its set destinations.

In this article, the attention will be on the key job compelling communication plays in the every day workings of a nursing organization. We will begin by taking a look at the significance of successful communication from various points and proceed to look at its significance as well as how it tends to be accomplished in business.

Taking a look at the Meaning of Effective Communication from Different Angles

A definitive objective of each type of communication - up close and personal meeting, phone call, remote communication, videoconferencing, talking with, email, letter or memo - is to get a normal reaction in the type of input from the beneficiary to the sender. This is the thing that viable communication is all about. It is tied in with guaranteeing that the data is well-bundled and appropriately transmitted, so the beneficiary comprehends the message and reacts emphatically. As it were, viable communication is the one that accomplishes the outcomes for which it is proposed.

Communication can be taken a look at from various angles, for example, the method of articulation (oral or composed, or even non-verbal correspondence), the reason for the communication, the group of spectators, the data stream (vertical, flat or askew), and so forth. Communication can be inward (inside the organization) or outer (with lower down entities). It can likewise be relational or mass communication; relational when it includes two individuals and a group when it requires meetings, discourses, symposia, and workshops. There is likewise mass communication which has to do with speaking with the majority via types such as radio, the TV, the newspaper, the Web, and so forth.). From whichever point it is seen, communication must be viewed as successful when it brings about the ideal input.

Oral communication includes the utilization of verbally expressed words and could appear as eye to eye discussions, talking with someone, phone calls, voice message, meetings, group dialogs, oral guidelines, remote communication, videoconferencing, and so forth. Oral correspondence is snappy and grants prompt criticism just as quick reaction does to input. Members can pose inquiries and get prompt explanations. In addition, motion and outward appearance can be utilized to strengthen the expected message. The restrictions of oral communication incorporate weakness to blunders and error and absence of changelessness.

Written communication, as the name suggests, includes using composed words. It can come in the forms of nursing letters, memoranda, reports, minutes of meetings, written discourses, and so on. Written communication has the benefits of correction before transmission, perpetual quality and its availability for reference purposes. It additionally diminishes the danger of mutilation in importance; hence, it tends to be considered as a perfect mechanism for long and complex messages which, whenever handed-off orally travel through many mediators, and it can undoubtedly be misshaped or misjudged.

Another favorable position of written medium is it can easily be duplicated in many ways (for example photocopying) and disseminated to numerous beneficiaries. One of its significant confinements is postponed input; the perusing of long records might exhaust and the composition of an answer could likewise be deferred by various other components. Written communication likewise does not have the nearness of motion, outward appearance and different types of non-verbal communication fit for strengthening significance in communication.

The decision of the mode of communication relies upon the idea of the message to be transmitted. As previously seen, while written medium is the ideal mode for exchanges that require changeless documentation, the oral medium is perfect for messages that require quick criticism.

One needs to consider the conditions so they can decide if to utilize a phone call, an up close and personal meeting, an email, a written and marked record, and so on. The elements to be viewed as well as when picking the mechanism of correspondence include: desperation, convention, danger of distortion, classification, legitimate ramifications or the requirement for future reference, the nature and size of the group of spectators, and so forth.

Communication in nursing is generally proposed to accomplish explicit purposes, for example, giving information, making a request, giving clarification, influence, consolation, making exchanges, and so forth. Communicating to illuminate is many times a demonstration of presenting, telling, declaring or announcing; it is normally planned for advising individuals about new product offerings, costs, names, addresses, and so on.

If the reason for communication is to bring about something, the message must be bundled with the end goal of moving the group of spectators to action by the utilization of words. This kind of communication is perfect for publicizing an item or persuading workers.

At the point when communication is only for nursing transactions, for example, contracts, understandings, receipts, and so on, the message must be bundled such that gives no space for distortion or legitimate activities. In this sort of communication, the accentuation is on the exactness and propriety of the given data, for example, the date of exchange, the concurred terms and conditions, the concurred costs, the complete total and money, names, locations and marks of meetings to the understanding, and so forth. The fact being made here is that, in order to accomplish successful communication, the message must be bundled to fill the particular need as well as the specific event of communication.

Step by step instructions to Ensure Effective Communication in Business

Note that poor or insufficient correspondence is in charge of a circumstance where the beneficiary doesn't comprehend what the person in question has perused or heard and along these lines can't give any constructive input. This infers the sign of powerful correspondence is a well-bundled and appropriately transmitted message - that is, a message that is equipped for drawing in the beneficiary's reaction in type of positive input.

Language ought to be viewed as the most significant type of compelling correspondence. The communicator must guarantee that the language the individual uses is clear, exact and fitting to the group of spectators, reason and event for which the message is proposed. The utilization of casual language where an amiable and formal register is required, for example, can render the message incapable. Longwindedness or the utilization of superfluously complex developments can just make space for distortion; thus the abbreviation 'KISS': Keep it short and straightforward.

Likewise, the utilization of articulations, languages and trendy expressions that the crowd is new to can exhibit obstructions to them and therefore upset correspondence. Where specialized language and terms are utilized, they should be characterized and clarified as per the information of the crowd. Whatever is the motivation behind the correspondence, the communicator must interface with the crowd by utilizing clear and exact language and expelling each type of uncertainty or boundary so the group of spectators can have a full comprehension of the message.

Successful correspondence is best accomplished when the reason or focal thought of the message is expressed plainly and the subordinate thoughts adequately recognized and identified with the primary reason in a normally persuading way. Ensure that the material is organized in a sensible and rational request, with each passage containing just a single principle thought that is plainly expressed and upheld with significant, adequate and influential focuses. To accomplish lucidness, new data must be connected to recently talked about data in a manner that draws in the peruser and strengthens the central matters. The finish of the message must rehash the primary reason and determine the move to be made.

Guaranteeing accuracy or linguistically is likewise an essential part of compelling correspondence, since ungrammaticality is fit for misshaping meaning or undermining believability, in this manner preventing correspondence. It is critical to guarantee that guidelines of language and grammar are pursued, that right words are utilized to pass on the planned significance and that accentuation reflects standard utilization. At long last, the whole work must be edited to guarantee that the last duplicate is free of mechanical mistakes.

Most importantly, it ought to be noticed that the reason for nursingcommunication is, in expansive terms, purchasing and selling. Nursingcommunication is more often than not about handy issues, for example, items, costs, limits, deals, conveyance, installments, etc. The fruitful businessperson is one who accomplishes his objectives, and to accomplish his objectives, he should impart adequately through clearness of articulation. He needs to display his messages to his crowds in the most clear and most direct way.

Correspondence is a basic piece of regular day to day existence. A few people are normally greater at conveying than others and some increasingly experienced. In the event that we are great at talking, notwithstanding, we shouldn't be tricked into accepting that we are great at conveying. In like manner, on the off chance that we happen to be tranquil, that doesn't mean we are terrible communicators.

All that we do throughout everyday life, and at work, imparts a message to other people. Furthermore, in an influential position, it is essential to ensure we are imparting the correct message. Powerful correspondence is in this way one of the most significant administration abilities.

The greater part of us have likely heard this platitude:

"It's not what we state but rather how we state it."

This can be valid; as powerful communicators, in any case, we ought to get that:

"It is the thing that we state and how, when,

where and why we state it."

What, how, when, where and why we convey is the distinction among negative and positive communications, circumstances, results and connections. It very well may be the key contrast between being a poor head and an uncommon pioneer.

Having the right stuff to convey adequately is one of the keys to driving individuals viably.

Viable correspondence is a difficult and complex procedure as there is consistently the potential for misconception.

How about we consider, for instance, the inquiry: "Who settled on that choice?"

The inquiry "Who settled on that choice?" appears to be a clear question, anyway relying upon who asked it, how they asked it, who was asked and under what conditions it was solicited there could be any number from astonishing reactions (either spoken or thought, for example,

"Goodness that'd be correct - I've toiled over this for a considerable length of time independent from anyone else and just now you choose to descend here and get included!"

or on the other hand

"I did and if it's not impeccable I don't have opportunity to fix it; I have considerably more significant things to do!"

Imagine a scenario where the full question was.

"Who settled on that choice - it looks phenomenal! What an extraordinary thought!"

On the off chance that the inquiry had been conveyed along these lines, all things considered, a considerably more positive reaction would have been gotten.

This model exhibits that correspondence can

be exceptionally testing, which is actually why, so as to be powerful pioneers, we have to figure out how to convey adequately.

So where do we start?

There are many, numerous features to successful correspondence, for example, utilizing and translating non-verbal communication, accepting analysis decidedly, emphatic correspondence and overseeing correspondence hindrances, just to give some examples.

As a beginning stage, here are three of the most significant successful relational abilities to consider:

1. Think about their point of view

Viable correspondence isn't about us and it's not just about imparting our message; it is additionally about understanding the planned importance of the other individual's message.

Our correspondence goal is 'to accomplish shared regard and comprehension'.

This implies when we are speaking with somebody, we have to try to consider the message they are conveying to us (both verbally and non-verbally) from their point of view. On the off chance that we take the data we are getting and think about it as far as:

- what is critical to them
- what their needs are
- what their favored method for conveying is
- how they are feeling, and
- what their conditions are

... we stand a vastly improved possibility of accomplishing our correspondence objective, 'shared regard and comprehension.

2. Constructive reframes

Listening is seemingly the most fundamental aptitude for successful correspondence and is an unquestionably more troublesome procedure than simply hearing the words somebody is stating.

Viable listening includes centering our ears, eyes and psyches on the speaker and the blend of verbal and non-verbal (non-verbal communication) messages they are conveying to us so as to increase a genuine comprehension of the point they are attempting to pass on.

We have to:

- shut out the contemplations that are coursing through our psyches (counting what we intend to state straightaway)

- overlook the outside action that might occur around us

... what's more, center around tuning in. Else we are probably going to miss a key sign that could assist us with understanding their message totally.

Figuring out how to impart emphatically and productively will quite often prompt improved results. To enable us to make our sentences increasingly positive and valuable, we can utilize Constructive Reframes. Valuable Reframes essentially include evacuating negative words in a sentence and including positive words.

How about we think about the accompanying negative sentence for instance:

"This report is garbage".

If we somehow managed to utilize a

Constructive Reframe, we could rather say:

"There are a few regions of this report could be improved".

In spite of the fact that we are as yet conveying a similar general message, the productive sentence is a lot simpler for the other individual to acknowledge. All things considered, they will tune in to our message as opposed to feel assaulted and become guarded.

Viable correspondence consistently begins with a message. A few chiefs battle with conveying their messages in a manner that is comprehendible to their devotees despite the fact that they accept there ought to be no confusions about the message. In all actuality, while individuals converse with each other consistently seeing language and correspondence as a simple ability, conveying a message as a pioneer necessitates that the message be customized to the devotee's inclinations. This can some of the time demonstrate to be a disagreeable and simple errand of the pioneer, however it is important to achieve so as to convey the most conceivable message with minimal space for inconstancy. The objective of conveying a message to a devotee ought to be to get them to act in the ideal way that the message speaks to. In the event that a pioneer needs their adherents to finish an assignment in a short measure of time, at that point they should convey their message one way. On the off chance that a pioneer needs their adherents to finish an assignment simply after another occasion has been finished, at that point they should convey their message another way. It is dependent upon the pioneer to convey their message in the manner they feel will impact their supporters the most which ought to pass on that an assignment must be finished in the precise manner the pioneer needs. On the off chance that that message is conveyed in the most ideal manner conceivable, at that point the pioneer ought to expect the best outcomes and their objectives happening as intended.

Framing the message

Since you have a message, the significant activity, as a pioneer, is to outline your message in a manner that is most persuasive to your adherents. There are numerous parts engaged with this progression including concentrating on the language, the idea, and the planning of the message. The language that is picked to speak to the message ought to be chosen in a fastidious manner. Language is a definitive apparatus for influence, so using compelling language while conveying a message will put pioneers in a position where adherents will be bound to tune in. Moreover, the language chose ought to be clear and self-evident. This will at last help explain the message that the pioneer wishes to convey in an understandable way and will likewise lift impact. Proceeding onward, thought of the message ought to be considered. In the event that a message is to be conveyed so adherents will acknowledge and grasp it, at that point a pioneer must place extraordinary idea by thinking about the inward encircling of that message. This is the place it is significant that pioneers use the psychological models of their message dependent on their basic objectives. It is critical to utilize thought and reflection to affirm that a message is as yet identified with its fundamental objectives and qualities. Doing so will take into consideration more congruency between the pioneer's character and the message they convey. Last, planning is something a pioneer should grasp since it will prove to be useful if off the cuff correspondence bringing out conditions ought to emerge. By making a decision about the potential inquiries that will be posed later on, pioneers can set themselves up to keep up congruency and abstain from conveying blended messages. By rehearsing planning, a pioneer ventures into the domain of being totally arranged to deal with any sort of circumstance that will either help or damage them when influencing others to pursue - however further dialog of this will come straightaway.

Preparing a spontaneous communication

The craft of surrounding can demonstrate hard for even the most experienced pioneer, in spite of the fact that the best heads have a sharp capacity to rehearse the procedure. Another expertise that pioneers should catch up on to assist them with thinking ahead is the utilization of preparing. Preparing, in correspondence, is an approach to enact esteems, missions, dreams, expectations, or potentially alluring language before correspondence even begins. While utilizing preparing as a system can appear to be marginally manipulative, it tends to be utilized for good too. The entire objective of utilizing preparing systems is to put a thought regarding a message before it is even conveyed. So as to do this, a pioneer must exhibit high qualities and spotlight on a specific setting. Devotees will start to acknowledge where the message might head and shape their very own sentiments or backing for the message before it is conveyed. While they are building up these conclusions, it is significant that the pioneer assesses and thinks about all parts of the message while cutting any ambiguities or remaining details so as to make flawless explanation when imparting the message. It is likewise a smart thought to get ready for unconstrained correspondence by considering all parts of the message just as possibilities that could create from the thought. It is smarter to cover oneself than to be ill-equipped and compromised of loss of trustworthiness or congruency. Keep in mind however, on the off chance that you are gotten stuck a tough situation, it is smarter to rehash your message with its hidden qualities boisterous and clear as opposed to faltering into obscure or undesired region just to have adherents rebate anything said later on. When the pioneer conveys the message, after the previous setting and thoughts, the devotees will be have shaped conclusions on the message, however they will be inside fulfilled that they "speculated" what the message would be. This is incredible provided that supporters concur with the pioneer, at that point they will indicate energy for anticipating what the pioneer would impart. In the event that they don't concur, at that point it really is great that the pioneer arranged for unconstrained correspondence before conveying the message.

Setting SENSITIVITY

With regards to conveying, actions speak louder than words, and tuning in to adherents, seeing how they think and what they expect will frequently put a pioneer on the correct way to convey a powerful message. Focusing on the setting of a circumstance previously, during, and in the wake of conveying a message is essential for progress. A pioneer should have the option to translate and assess a setting to affect the progression of correspondence when developing and showing their message. To do this, a pioneer ought to analyze logical impacts, their own penetrability, consistency, reality, and timing. This paper has officially addressed consistency and reality by clarifying the significance of binds messages to mental models and ensuring that the message is harmonious with qualities and objectives. It is likewise essential to look at the relevant impacts of adherents by dissecting their way of life and their qualities. What's more, a pioneer must be penetrable implying that they should have the option to grasp new thoughts, convictions, and practices. The administration world can regularly be sporadic, particularly when imparting messages to adherents, and pioneers should have the option to adjust to new circumstances by grasping new thoughts. Last, timing is one of the most significant and powerful devices of correspondence. Pioneers ought to realize when to discuss explicit pieces of a message and when to disguise different parts just to uncover the extra subtleties at a later and progressively fitting time. This doesn't imply that pioneers should conceal reality from their devotees. Rather, they should cautiously choose which parts of a message ought to be uncovered at specific occasions so as to develop to the best message deliverable. What sort of pioneer needs to demolish their amazements in any case?

Keep away from MIXED MESSAGES

With regards to conveying, actions speak louder than words, and tuning in to supporters, seeing how they think and what they expect will regularly put a pioneer on the correct way to convey a viable message. Focusing on the setting of a circumstance previously, during, and in the wake of conveying a message is essential for progress. A pioneer should have the option to decipher and assess a setting to affect the progression of correspondence when building and showing their message. To do this, a pioneer ought to inspect logical impacts, their own penetrability, consistency, reality, and timing. This paper has officially addressed consistency and reality by clarifying the significance of binds messages to mental models and ensuring that the message is harmonious with qualities and objectives. It is likewise imperative to inspect the relevant impacts of devotees by breaking down their way of life and their qualities. Moreover, a pioneer must be penetrable implying that they should have the option to grasp new thoughts, convictions, and practices. The authority world can regularly be sporadic, particularly when conveying messages to adherents, and pioneers should have the option to adjust to new circumstances by grasping new ideas. Last, timing is one of the most significant and viable instruments of correspondence. Pioneers ought to realize when to discuss explicit pieces of a message and when to hide different parts just to uncover the extra subtleties at a later and progressively suitable time. This doesn't imply that pioneers should conceal reality from their devotees. Rather, they should cautiously choose which parts of a message ought to be uncovered at specific occasions so as to develop to the best message deliverable. What sort of pioneer needs to demolish their amazements in any case?

Variety in Communication

Over and over, it appears that any hierarchical counsel makes reference to assorted variety some place. While it might sound extremely repetitive to approximately, one can't express how significant decent variety is in the work environment! The receptive methodology: managing claims, broken groups, work environment basic frequencies are all things enveloped by an absence of decent variety and can be maintained a strategic distance from with assorted variety preparing as well as other proactive methodologies revolved around decent variety. Other than sexism, ageism, and bigotry to give some examples, numerous other unfair convictions block execution. In correspondence alone, not understanding or perceiving alternate points of view can reduce execution procedures and results. What's more, undivided attention to one gathering of individuals or workers over others likewise raises numerous potential outcomes. Through decent variety preparing, compelling correspondence practices can be accomplished to ensure everybody in your association feels regarded and will perform to enable the association to succeed.

Incredible correspondence for nurse caretakers is a case of focal points given by a walkie talkie. They need a convenient gadget that will assist them with communicating in achieving their objective to deal with the patients. Nurse attendants need to utilize this gadget in certain condition when they are not permitted to have direct correspondence or up close and personal correspondence. By utilizing this specific specialized gadget, they will have the option to get in touch with one another without leaving the patients. You can get straightforward data from this article to enable you to get the best possible strides in utilizing walkie talkie for correspondence arrangement of nurse attendants.

In the first place, you have to set up your walkie talkies and furthermore clasps to enable the nurse caretakers to affix these gadgets on their regalia. You have to ensure that each nurse caretaker has walkie talkies in their grasp. Abstain from sharing the gadgets for a similar move and ensure that all gadgets are accessible to be reached. You likewise need to prepare them about the activity and the arrangement of walkie talkies. Tell them increasingly about the best approach to turn it on or off. They likewise should be prepared while in transit to change the recurrence or channel.

Obviously, investing more energy with patients isn't the appropriate response. The truth of the matter is, except if hindrances are evacuated and staffing and procedures improved, there is no more opportunity for nursing correspondence. Any proposal that nurse attendants ought to invest more energy - time that they don't have - is goading and breeds protection from progress techniques. Accordingly, it's useful to concentrate not on the amount of time attendants spend, yet on the nature of that time with their patients and families. The test is to verify that their minding goes over to the individuals they serve during the valuable time they do go through with them.

So in what capacity can nurse caretakers verify that their minding is felt by patients and families during the valuable time they go through with them?

In the event that I could propel one expertise in nursing correspondence that would make leaps forward in the patient experience and employment fulfillment, it would be the ability of "nearness." This learnable aptitude includes controlling your consideration so the individual on the less than desirable end feels like the focal point of your universe during the valuable minutes you have with them. The settlements: Patients feel your concentration and minding, you interface with them, and your work turns out to be progressively important. When you practice nearness, the patient feels significant - that they are your sole core interest. They additionally feel like your spirit center. This encourages them feel bolstered, less on edge and they really mend quicker. Additionally, when you are completely present, you don't miss significant signals about the individual's contemplations and emotions - prompts that help you address individuals' issues incredibly well.

Nursing assessment scale for relational abilities

This is a procedure by which the nurse attendants in the emergency clinic or the human services foundation are made a decision on their skills and practice. This judgment may include students, practice towards patient, their family and the relational abilities included and other clinical practice with respect to their work involvement.

More often than not the nursing assessment scale for relational abilities includes their exhibition and moving toward the patient. The decisions are impacted by the information gathered that is the particular data gathered by the patients execution by the attendant and the ends drawn towards the information gathered. The experts may gather similar information to assess the powerful results of the nurse attendant or nursing understudy.

There was an examination led for nursing assessment scale for relational abilities so as to set up a self assessment ECS (Empathic Understanding Scale) that would quantify compassion. This is the most significant factor for an attendant to build up a decent correspondence with the patient in the nursing clinical circumstance.

The advancement of this exploration of self

assessment or EUS depended on the empathic understanding scale assessed by others. In the past examination that was directed it was said that it is hard for a third individual to scale and assess a nurse caretakers understanding in the clinical nursing circumstance.

Nursing Informatics is the joining of clinical nursing with data the board and PC forms. It is a generally new concentration in human services that consolidates nursing abilities with data innovation mastery. Nurse attendant informatics pros oversee and convey nursing information and data to improve basic leadership by customers, patients, nurse attendants and other medicinal services suppliers.

The nursing procedure has four principle steps: arranging, execution, assessment, and appraisal. In any case, since data the executives is coordinated into the nursing procedure and practice, some nursing networks distinguish a fifth step in the nursing procedure: documentation. Documentation and patient-focused consideration are the center segments of the nursing procedure. Robotized documentation is indispensably significant, for nursing, yet though patient couldn't care less. Exceptional, exact data at each progression of the nursing procedure is the way to sheltered, astounding patient-focused consideration.

The fruitful execution of data frameworks in nursing and human services requires the accompanying: First, it is important to have all around structured frameworks that help the nursing procedure inside the way of life of an association. The subsequent prerequisite is having the acknowledgment and joining of data frameworks into the customary work process of the nursing procedure and patient consideration. At long last, it is critical to have assets that can bolster the recently referenced variables. One of the best and important assets a medicinal services association can include is a Nurse informatics masters.

Nursing Informatics Specialists

Nursing Informatics Specialists are master clinicians with a broad clinical practice foundation. These people have involvement in using and actualizing the nursing procedure. These nurse attendants have superb diagnostic and basic reasoning aptitudes. They additionally comprehend the patient consideration conveyance work process and combination focuses for robotized documentation. Having extra training and involvement with data frameworks is additionally significant for this occupation. At last, Nursing Informaticists are incredible undertaking administrators in view of the similitude between the venture the board procedure and the nursing procedure.

To be focused in this field one ought to get comfortable with social databases by taking a class about database structure. They ought to likewise end up equipped and OK with MS Office, particularly Excel, Access and Visio.

Why these occupations are Important to Healthcare?

Nurse attendant and wellbeing informatics carry a lot of significant worth to patients and the social insurance framework. A few instances of how they offer some incentive include:

Offer help to the nursing work procedures utilizing innovation

Expanding the exactness and culmination of nursing documentation

Improving the nurse caretaker's work process

Computerizing the gathering and reuse of nursing information

Encouraging investigation of clinical information

Giving nursing substance to institutionalized dialects

HIMSS and RHIO

To give some foundation on the field of

human services/nursing informatics, there are some overseeing bodies for this field. The Healthcare Information and Management Systems Society (HIMSS) is the principle administering body for medicinal services and nursing informatics experts. This gathering, framed in 2004, has the accompanying four objectives: NI mindfulness, training, assets (counting sites), and RHIO (Regional Health Information Organization).

RHIOs are otherwise called Community Health Information Networks (CHINs). These are the systems that associate doctors, emergency clinics, research centers, radiology focuses and protection companies. They all offer and transmit persistent data electronically through a safe framework. Those associations that are a piece of RHIOs have a nursinginterest in improving the nature of social insurance being regulated.

Steps to a Job in This Field

To go into the nursing informatics field,

commonly you need at least a multi year degree. There are explicit wellbeing informatics degrees accessible. Gaining your Bachelor's of Science in Nursing (BSN) is likewise a necessity before sitting for the ANCC confirmations test for Nursing Informatics. A few people start with only a multi year degree or confirmation, however proceed to win their BSN before getting to be affirmed. Despite the fact that there are a few distinct courses for getting into the field, the most supported way is to gain a Master's in Nursing Informatics from the beginning, in any case, most people start their profession before procuring their graduate degree.

Most nurse caretakers who are in the informatics field start in a forte region, for example, the Intensive Care Unit (ICU), Perioperative Services (OR), Med-Surg, Orthopedic Nursing, or Oncology, just to give some examples, and work in that claim to fame field for an all-encompassing period. Working in a forte territory encourages nurse attendants become more acquainted with the typical working procedures and schedules just as comprehend the patient consideration process in their strength. They as a rule are specialists at their forte and afterward create interests in mechanized documentation or some other innovative medicinal services center. They at that point will in general slowly move into a data frameworks clinical help job.

Nursing informatics is the mix of clinical nursing abilities with some PC procedures and abnormal state data the executives. Nursing informatics is a totally new perspective in the human services industry and capacities with the mix of nursing aptitudes and mechanical skill. The masters in this field are required to keep up nursing information. They are additionally expected to impart any data that can ad lib and pace basic leadership by patients, attendants and different customers and social insurance suppliers.

The way toward nursing includes four distinct advances. These are arranging, execution, perception and evaluation.

Nonetheless, since data the executives is joined with the way toward nursing and furthermore with its training, a couple of nursing networks have included another progression in the process that is known as documentation. At the point when concentrated profoundly, the documentation and explicit patient-focused consideration have been distinguished as the principle job players in nursing forms. Robotized documentation is basic, and for nursing, yet for each patient consideration framework. Refreshed and exact data about the patient at each degree of nursing can be the best approach to verify and better quality patient consideration.

There are a couple of things that should be done in social insurance and nursing offices for the fruitful execution of the data framework. Fundamentally, it is basic to have great, explicitly planned frameworks that can deal with the nursing framework in an association. Furthermore, however of equivalent significance, is the acknowledgment and appropriate combination of the recently introduced data framework into the typical work process. At long last, the association should likewise have appropriate assets that can keep up the previously mentioned two elements. Nurse attendant informatics pros are the best that a nursing office or an emergency clinic can get with regards to control nursing informatics.

What are nursing informatics pros?

These pros can be considered as master clinicians that have a broad foundation in clinical practices. Nursing informatics authorities are experienced experts who have used and actualized the nursing procedure. These nurse attendants have basic deduction abilities just as high expository aptitudes. The nurse caretakers are likewise able to comprehend the conveyance work process of patient consideration and along these lines can discover better coordination focuses for the procedure of computerized documentation. Consequently, it very well may be said that nursing informatics pros are the best venture chiefs since they are the connection between the nursing procedure and undertaking the board procedure.

The right staff

As human life span keeps on expanding at a bewildering pace, we are living longer and more advantageous lives, being fit and dynamic even a very long time past our retirement. It might be difficult for us to accept that, at some point, we might be unequipped for dealing with ourselves. In any case, the maturing procedure is tireless and, on the off chance that we live into our 90s and past, may happen over numerous years. It's unavoidable that a huge level of seniors will in the long run need assistance or something to that affect in their everyday exercises.

Frequently, relatives can take in seniors who can never again live freely, or some kind of home-care game plan can be worked out. Notwithstanding, numerous seniors will in the long run need the full scope of administrations offered by a nursing home. Furthermore, there are such a large number of decisions accessible, choosing the correct nursing home turns into an essential choice. Look at every office that you are thinking about altogether, and pose a ton of inquiries.

In the first place, ensure that the office is in consistence with the majority of your state's permitting necessities. Discover what these prerequisites are, and ensure that any essential licenses are noticeably posted in the office. Additionally, get some information about the staff: what number of authorized enrolled nurse caretakers (RNs) are at the office at some random time? What different accreditations do staff individuals have? In the event that the senior that you are planning to put in the office has any uncommon needs or is experiencing a specific conditions, is the nursing staff prepared to adapt to these particular conditions?

Get some information about social administrations at the office: there ought to be a Social Services Worker on the staff to enable new occupants to change into the nursing home. The office ought to keep up an "Occupant's Bill of Rights"; request to see this, if accessible. Are inhabitants with specific conditions, for example, dementia, assembled in one wing, or are occupants spread around paying little heed to unique needs or conditions? More often than not, occupants want to associate with different seniors whose necessities and abilities are comparable.

Clearly, the office ought to be perfect and, while it ought not be boisterous, it ought not be totally quiet either. Ensure the foundation clamor level is suitable. Furthermore, attempt to visit during a feast time, so you can measure the nature of the nourishment. What do suppers comprise of? Could unique eating regimens be given if important?

Investigate the foundation. There ought to be smoke alarms, fire quenchers, and obviously stamped crisis exits. Is it simple to move around along the hallways? Passageways ought to be wide enough for wheelchairs to pass each other effectively, and restrooms obviously ought to be completely outfitted with wide spaces and handle rails. It ought to be simple for a senior utilizing a walker or wheelchair to move around openly.

Attempt to evaluate the general feeling of the office. Do the occupants and staff coexist well with each other; do the staff realize the inhabitants by name? Do the inhabitants have all the earmarks of being alert, very much prepared, and clean? Are the rooms new? Each floor ought to have its own clothing office, and materials ought to be changed regularly. Different comforts may incorporate a bank, a blessing shop, or a hair salon.

Additionally, get some information about recreational exercises. How frequently are exercises given, and how are they regulated? Is there an activity program and a health specialist on staff? Exercise gear ought to be anything but difficult to utilize, and proper for seniors. There might be extraordinary regions for PC use, reflection, artworks and games, and perusing; is there a library? Would residents be able to go outside - is there a nursery zone outside, with trails proper for wheelchairs?

On the off chance that your senior has extraordinary needs, get some information about close to home consideration programs, including restoration (from stroke, for example). In the event that there are no prepared physical advisors on staff, ensure that you can organize to have a specialist come as expected to work with your senior.

What's more, obviously, you should get some answers concerning costs. Medicare and customary nurse coverage for the most part doesn't cover long haul nursing home consideration, so examine the choices in detail. Maybe your senior has long haul care protection, or can fit the bill for Medicaid. Else, you may need to spend down assets to meet all requirements for Medicaid.

Make certain to look at in any event a couple of offices in your general vicinity, to get some reason for examination. Given the scope of decisions, you will positively discover a nursing home that is helpful and reasonable for your motivations.

Nobody appreciates the way toward finding a nursing home for their cherished one, yet when their wellbeing is decaying before their eyes, the opportunity may have arrived to locate the correct nursing home for them. There are four stages that you might need to pursue when considering nursing homes for the ones you cherish:

The initial step that you have to take when settling on the best nursing home is basically deciding if one is important. In the event that you see that your cherished one is getting more fit or encountering memory misfortune, you ought to have the person in question assessed by a geriatrician. The specialist will survey whether they can dress themselves, eat, without help, or in the event that they falls as often as possible. The doctor will likewise check for early indications of dementia.

On the off chance that the assessment discovers that a house is essential, you have to order a rundown of nursing homes to consider.

A few things you should search for are:

- Distance from you. You don't need your adored one to feel disengaged from their family, and you can keep an eye on the nature of consideration they are getting.

- History of consideration quality. You need to check for nursing homes that have a higher positioning, while at the same time remembering that these will be the most looked for after, and will probably have a holding up rundown. You can discover this data on state wellbeing division sites.

- Keep check of the parental figures and their calendars. The more parental figures that a home has, the more noteworthy the probability that it will have better care.

- Find a supporter. This individual will think about the different nursing homes, and may likewise enable you to show signs of improvement ones. They will likewise realize where to go to locate the vital data on each nursing home's consideration and wellbeing.

The following thing you ought to do is visit every one of the finalists. While you are visiting, the directors addresses that are custom fitted to the requirements of your adored one. You ought to likewise fluctuate your visits to various days and times. Things to search for are a full parking garage, the hints of guests, how the staff identifies with the patients, how the inhabitants play and eat, and undesirable scents.

At long last, when you have moved your adored one into their new home, you have to visit every so often with the goal that you can screen their consideration. You ought to anticipate an alteration period while your adored one becomes accustomed to the new environment. During these visits make note of any progressions to your adored one's wellbeing, air, and appearance. On the off chance that you see any issues, tranquilly carry it to the consideration of the managers, as it might be something that they didn't know about.

Numerous grown-up offspring of senior guardians today face a troublesome issue. Better nourishment and different therapeutic advances have prompted individuals living longer than at any other time, yet as a rule, it's not prudent for senior residents to live alone. Seniors that experience the ill effects of dementia or have an ailment that requires close checking, just as those with versatility weaknesses, may confront hazardous living conditions whenever left alone in their homes. Others may basically not be open to living alone, might be not able stay aware of the cooking or home upkeep, or may locate that a powerlessness to drive hampers their capacity to live freely. There are numerous alternatives for these seniors and their families. Some grown-up youngsters arrange day by day visits to their maturing guardian's home, while others move in with their parent or move the parent into their own home. Contracting in-home consideration is constantly a well known alternative, and obviously, numerous individuals pick nursing offices for their friends and family.

Moving a maturing guardian into a nursing office is constantly a troublesome choice for a grown-up tyke, and numerous individuals have just an ambiguous thought of what these offices resemble or ought to resemble before they start the arrangement procedure. It's a smart thought to realize what to search for when thinking about different nursing offices. Remember that the individual who will live in the office ought to consistently be associated with the choice to the degree that they're able to do.

When picking a nursing office, you should visit in any event three or four of them, if not more, before you start to settle on a choice. Various offices offer various degrees of consideration and administration, so make certain to concentrate your pursuit on offices that are most proper for your parent's needs. Is your parent for the most part equipped for autonomous living, yet needing transportation administrations, light housekeeping, and a close by restorative staff if there should be an occurrence of crisis? Assuming this is the case, at that point a helped living office might be a suitable decision. You can discover these as independent offices or regarding a nursing home offering talented consideration, where your parent can be moved should their condition decay. In the event that your parent is experiencing dementia, you should search for a nursing home that has a protected dementia ward with staff prepared in thinking about dementia patients. A ceaseless disease may require a nursing office with a talented consideration wing.

When you're visiting nursing homes, focus on the consider lights that are normally situated over the rooms. Nursing offices are ordinarily staffed by nurse attendants, nurture assistants, and various help and authoritative staff, every one of whom can answer an inhabitants call ringer. A call ringer ought to never take over a moment or two to react to. In the event that you see consider lights that stay on for over a moment or two during the hour of your visit, be attentive. This might be an indication that the house is understaffed, or that the standard of consideration isn't up to where you need it to be.

You ought to likewise observe the inhabitants that you find in the corridors and regular regions. It is anything but a decent sign on the off chance that you don't perceive any inhabitants in these zones during a daytime visit; that implies that they are sleeping or in their rooms rather than up and occupied with exercises. It's additionally not a decent sign on the off chance that you see an enormous number of them lounging around and sitting idle. During the day, you should see many nursing home occupants up and alert, wearing road garments with clean faces and brushed hair, and partaking in exercises or associating with different inhabitants.

At last, focus on your nose. A nursing home, similar to an emergency clinic, is a restorative office and may smell marginally germ-free, and the periodic awful aroma is not out of the ordinary. Be that as it may, a foul scent ought to surely not saturate the spot, nor should it smell as though somebody splashed loads of deodorizer so as to cover a terrible scent. Sustenance should smell appealing, inhabitants' skin and hair should smell clean, and the rooms should smell new also.

On the off chance that your older adored one needs consistent consideration and you just don't have opportunity important to give the person in question the consideration they need, you might look nursing homes as a possibility for help. There are an assortment of rules to remember when you are visiting potential offices for your friends and family. Each spot will have its own special qualities, and it is dependent upon you to figure out which are most significant with regards to the consideration and the wellbeing of your relative.

With regards to first taking a gander at the potential outcomes for nursing homes for your adored one, you might be a piece overpowered from the outset. There are numerous subtleties to analyze. When you are discovering which spots to call, talk with a confirmations agent to plan a gathering to view to put. During your gathering, focus on how you are being treated by the staff, and remember the treatment of your friends and family. Initial introductions are very significant. From the staff to the entryway and the conveniences, focus on everything about.

On the off chance that you see other individuals who right now live in these nursing homes, basically start up a discussion with them. Ask them inquiries, for example, to what extent they've lived there, how they feel about their treatment, etc. Individual suggestions from companions of current inhabitants can likewise be useful in your journey. All through your visit, don't be bashful to pose the same number of inquiries as you might want. Pay heed to how the individuals around you are communicating. Talk with different representatives or inhabitants while you are there to discover how agreeable and welcoming activities are.

When review the inhabitant's rooms in a home, observe how roomy or welcoming the room is. Space is a significant perspective to consider. Envision your adored one living in the specific space to check whether the person would feel good. It is significant that they see their new home as welcoming, and less like an emergency clinic room and progressively like a room.

You ought to likewise remember the enhancements and recreational choices. Are there any exercises continuing during your visit? How are inhabitants welcomed to take an interest in these exercises? Are exercises and get-togethers ones that your adored one would need to take an interest in?

When experiencing distinctive nursing homes, there are an assortment of choices to look over, and the pursuit may not be the most effortless. Do your examination before you go on your visits. It is basic that you pick the correct alternative for your cherished one, so doing record verifications and going to see them for yourself is very significant.

Remaining at a nursing and recovery focus is

distressing, however picking an inside shouldn't be. With the best possible information, assessing places for the correct characteristics turns out to be simple. Being sentenced to a low quality nursing and recovery focus exacerbates the worry of avoiding home. Early research enables families to keep away from this issue.

Start with the administration's evaluating framework for nursing and restoration focuses. The Centers for Medicare and Medicaid Services assess the country's focuses and allocates a star rating to every one. Appraisals depend on wellbeing assessment information, quality measures, and staffing and extend from one star to five. Homes with three or less stars ought to be stayed away from if at all conceivable.

Visits from loved ones keep patients rationally stable. An inside ought to be near friends and family to encourage visits. The best care accessible won't be sufficient for a patient who gets no close to home visits. It might be ideal to pick a four star focus near family over a five star focus situated far away. Guarantee that the meeting hours work for the potential guests. An office that confines visits to times when none of the patient's companions are accessible probably won't be the best decision.

Visiting a nursing and recovery focus face to face is the most significant advance. A middle ought to have a perfect, systematic appearance and a charming smell. Nursing staff ought to be neighborly and collaborating with patients. Rooms ought to be enormous and embellished with patients' belongings. In the event that patients who appear as though they need assistance are left sitting unattended, that is a major warning. Converse with a portion of the patients that appear to be anxious to talk. They can offer bits of knowledge to how the consideration in the office truly is.

Long haul care ombudsmen are autonomous government laborers doled out to screen nursing and recovery focuses. Objections and compliments about focuses are coordinated to ombudsmen. In the wake of finding a strategically placed focus with a high star rating and a solid exhibition during an in-person visit, reaching the inside's ombudsman gives a goal supposition. An ombudsman will think about protests that may not be promptly obvious, or know about pending administration changes.

CHAPTER TWO

A nurse background skills

Nurse attendants are patient backers. To turn into a fruitful and viable nurse attendant, you don't just need to secure the vital instruction and licenses to rehearse however you additionally need to gangs certain characteristics and abilities to enable you to perform in this quick paced industry. Nursing is an extremely requesting activity physically, rationally, inwardly, and mentally. Responsibility and commitment is an absolute necessity in each attendant.

Enthusiastic Skills

More often than not, nurse caretakers are encompassed with patients who need care. Other than therapeutic treatment, patients need enthusiastic help from their parental figures. Consequently, it is fundamental for nurse caretakers to mind, understanding and non judgmental. As a nurse caretaker, you will manage individuals from varying backgrounds; newborn children, teenagers, grown-ups and the older. You will likewise be treating patients from various social standings, race, religion and sexual direction.

Contingent upon the sort of office you are working in, you should think about individuals who are extremely wiped out, physically tested, or individuals who are experiencing distinctive physical, enthusiastic and mental issues. To be a successful nurse caretaker, you need to figure out how to relate to your patients and not get excessively sincerely appended or engaged with them or their conditions. Else, it will influence your exhibition and levelheadedness with regards to overseeing care and treatment.

Scholarly Skills

The nursing calling expects you to gain and hold a lot of data. As a nurse attendant, you should be shrewd, sorted out and you must have great performing multiple tasks aptitudes as you should play out different errands in a constrained measure of time. You should assemble and observe precise data about your patient's therapeutic history, course of treatment, and you will likewise need to deal with various supplies and drugs.

A decent foundation in science and math will be of incredible assistance as nurse attendants regularly should perform transformations on portions and will likewise be presented to microorganisms and infections.

Relational abilities

To appropriately carry out your responsibility

as a nurse attendant, you should speak with specialists and associates in a quick paced condition. You need great understanding abilities with the goal that specialists and nurse attendant supervisors don't have to rehash directions. Other significant aptitudes in correspondence that are important in the nursing calling are the capacity to communicate in and comprehend various dialects and gesture based communication.

Observational Skills

Specialists are occupied and patients have different concerns beside their ailments. Being perceptive is a significant trademark you should have so as to be a fruitful nurse caretaker. You ought to have the option to tell if a patient is experiencing issues regardless of whether the patient isn't whining. You ought to rush to see if something isn't right particularly in a patient's conduct.

Physical Skills

Nursing is physically requesting. Because of lack of nurse caretakers, they are frequently required to render extra long stretches of work. Some even labor for 36 hours in a row, contingent upon the prerequisite of the clinic. This is particularly valid in emergency clinics that are essentially understaffed. The greater part of all, you are around wiped out individuals more often than not and this makes you vulnerable to contaminations and illnesses. You must be physically fit so as to fulfill the physical needs of this activity.

The idea of Human Resources Development and Training is tied in with furnishing workers with the devices to build up their insight, individual aptitudes, hierarchical gifts and capacities. It can incorporate preparing, tutoring, nonappearance the board, progression arranging, HR training, distinguishing representatives with specific abilities or potential, nonattendance the executives, legitimization, execution the board and furthermore essential hierarchical improvement.

Basically the object of the activity is to boost the capability of a workforce of a limited size so as to make the best and productive administration ability that can be accomplished the situation being what it is.

Arrangement of HR Development and Training can be inside or outer, or in reality a program could include a mix of the two. As a rule an outer supplier will be appointed to start procedures, recognize squander and slackage inside the association, achieve some "fast successes" which will be valuable for resourcing the rest of the work that should be attempted, at that point inevitably to pull back and enable the association to keep on streamlining itself and create.

One other significant part of Human Resource Development, on the other hand referred to just as HRD, is to guarantee the ideal synchronization of individual abilities and gifts with the corporate needs of an association.

It is nothing unexpected that Human

Resources Development and Training has turned into an industry in its very own right, and their expert suppliers themselves utilize enormous quantities of individuals to offer exhortation and help to different organizations. One basic part of their work is to deal with any sentiments of doubt or trepidation that may be prompted by their essence just as to attempt to get the workforce "on side" so as to verify its co-activity for the span of the rearrangement time frame.

One method for empowering this to happen is through HR workshops, which help to reduce any secret that may be related with the work engaged with streamlining a corporate venture and improving its proficiency. HR courses can be offered which shape the attitude just as the real physical abilities for realizing hierarchical change.

Great chiefs will consistently comprehend that the expense of supplanting experienced staff and after that preparation their substitutions can be extensive, and this additionally gets its wake the threat of a further negative impact upon the resolve of the workforce. It is normally better and simpler to furnish existing staff with the correct abilities through which to understand their potential, and to make a situation that creates pride and responsibility with the base of interest upon assets.

In the initial segment of this article we examined the differentiation between an Influencing Paradigm, and a Service Paradigm, to promoting your instructing business. We talked about how showcasing your business is both morally substantial and industrially urgent, and how promoting is a basic procedure in accomplishing your training goal of positively affecting the lives of others.

To rapidly infer, we clarified that individuals with an Influencing Paradigm outlook see showcasing to be 'driving' and 'salesy.' They originate from the worldview that by advertising you are proactively impacting somebody in their choices. Or on the other hand explicitly that you may cause somebody to accomplish something they would not generally do.

Individuals from the Service Paradigm way of thinking acknowledge that prospects are individuals that have recognized for themselves their need to conjure change. Also, they've distinguished that a mentor will help them roll out that improvement. They perceive that the prospect has made the scholarly connect between their needs and how they need those should be satisfied.

To be an effective mentor, or in actuality fruitful in any business, it's important that you grasp a Service Paradigm outlook toward your promoting.

In this article we will further investigate precisely how you can build up a Service Paradigm advertising mentality.

Before we can start to examine how you can build up your Service Paradigm attitude, how about we take a gander at a portion of the attributes. Mentors with a Service Paradigm perceive that to help customers meet their goals, they have to:

- Recognize that everybody in business is in the matter of showcasing. Without customers they'll have nobody to convey their administrations as well and henceforth nobody to help.

- Actively advance their administrations through convincing publicizing that obviously depicts what they can offer customers.

- Ethically advance their administrations with watchfulness.

- Recognize the cycle of life of their prospects and routinely advance their administrations for whatever length of time that prospects permit.

- Understand that hello are regularly in a better position of information than find out what their customer needs to help them accomplish their objectives.

- Be empathic to the necessities of customers and effectively offer answers for them through different items and administrations.

- Value their customer's insight and basic leadership capacity.

- Not pre-empt their customer's needs and thus limit the range and extent of items and administrations they offer them.

- Always goes about as a moral consultant.

Service Paradigm promoting outlook

As a mentor, to outmaneuver your rivals you should make a specialty; and to assemble a fruitful business you should accomplish a Service Paradigm promoting outlook.

To build up your Service Paradigm advertising mentality:

1. Be resolved to succeed. You should be

completely confirmed that you will succeed. On the off chance that you simply need to succeed, however you're not willing to go the additional mile, you'll get cleared aside by those that are increasingly decided. In the event that you are really decided, you'll be sure and this certainty will naturally appear in your business and be straightforward to imminent customers, peers and the overall population. Imminent customers will need to be related with you, and customers will need to proceed with their association.

2. Endure. Mentors with an advertising attitude hold onto challenges as a major aspect of life and part of business. On the off chance that you see difficulties as obstructed hindrances you'll never build up a showcasing outlook. It's significant you acknowledge you will stand up to obstacles as a component of business. How you see these obstacles, as circumstances or obstructions, will radically impact your degree of progress. Steadiness is a key fixing in building up a showcasing mentality.

3. Stay positive. Truly nothing crushes an advertising mentality in excess of a negative frame of mind. A promoting outlook is a 'can do' disposition. Looked with a similar test, the mentor with a positive 'can do' advertising mentality will discover a way; the mentor with a pessimist frame of mind will submit and fall flat.

4. Set Goals. As a mentor this is something you should know a ton about. Set yourself explicit, reachable, stretch objectives.

5. Plan a procedure. Build up a particular strategy to accomplish your objectives. Distinguish what assets you'll require and the potential difficulties you may stand up to.

6. Actualize your arrangement. This is the most troublesome part. Usage of your arrangement. Alter it where required, change your objectives as others are achieved, adjust your arrangement if imperfections are seen, however consistently keep actualizing. Non-activity is the forerunner of business disappointment. On the off chance that you

keep on actualizing, your business will consistently continue forward force. On the off chance that you have energy, your heading (objectives and plans) can generally be balanced.

7. Continue advertising. Your prosperity or disappointment depends on your advertising. Continuously keep up your promoting mentality. Continuously be focussed on showcasing. It's a typical snare to become involved with the everyday 'activity' of your business and set advertising aside. This is a catastrophe waiting to happen. How viably you market will be the most compelling determinant on the achievement (or something else) of your business. Promoting isn't troublesome or befuddling, however it requires noteworthy continuous constancy and consideration. The minute you lose center around promoting your business is the minute your business execution will endure.

CHAPTER THREE

Develop good coaching mindset

What is having an amazing training mentality? To begin with, you should comprehend that there is a reasonable and clear contrast between an advisor and a specialist. Advisors are specialists, rehearsing and sharpening their aptitudes in the field. As a business mentor, you become the master. YOU help the customer explore the slippery territory while enabling that individual to pick the most perfectly awesome seminar all alone. As the magnificent business mentor you really join forces with the customer to help complete errands in an auspicious, proficient design. This aides hugely by structure the fundamental trust to fortify and stay your mentor customer relationship.

In the instructing procedure, you enable space for the customer to utilize his/her own imaginative procedure to shoulder natural product as self-disclosure. You accomplish this by being a specialist audience, utilizing your empathic listening abilities to see, instead of react. This makes a "security zone" for the customers to open up their own personalities and make their own answers.

Rather than turning into the "chief," or the donkey taking every necessary step for them, you are the companion strolling alongside them. The expert mentor figures out how to rapidly move trust by listening completely without any plans. Figure out how to regard the other individual as your OPW, or just individual on the planet. Be delayed to pass judgment, don't race to tackle, and give them space to be what their identity is. Training is designation in its preeminent structure.

In figuring out how to be a magnificent mentor, you should figure out how to conserve the time it takes accomplishing the errand. Be a functioning member by cooperating with your customers as opposed to be a better than them. This will enable you to reinforce their certainty and trust in you, ten times. Building up the vital abilities and solid mentality of expert mentors will limit your outstanding task at hand since you gather from your colleagues, customers, prospects, and expert partners, what the errands really are, with tremendous proficiency.

As an expert mentor, you should recognize what the hidden issues are. Regularly it is what isn't said that is generally noteworthy. As the expert mentor, you should figure out how to turn into an a lot further audience. It is an ability you should rehearse so as to turn into an ace audience and mentor. You can utilize these aptitudes in any of your connections, individual or expert, and take them to an a lot higher level.

Ensure the message you send is a similar message gotten. To discover the state and phase of the customer's matter of fact, you should put yourself in the other individual's shoes. Tune in to what's been going on in their lives, what moves they have made, who they course with, what their present foundation is, anything to give you a setting on how they may get your message. You will have the option to check out what your customers do and say as it were, utilizing your intuitive personality, building up your abilities and mentalities. Figure out how to perceive what is and isn't there. Most may not, be that as it may, anybody can apply this expertise. You should figure out how to have an all around prepared eye to separate the requirements in the entirety of your connections.

What activities would you be able to begin executing right away?

Start with rehearsing genuine listening shills-whether you are talking with a customer or relative, partner, or companion, work on being totally "at the time with them." Listen to comprehend, not to react. Come into their lounge rooms. Tune in for tones, speed, and delays. They are the signs along the street to tell you what's truly going on.

Feel what they are stating and NOT saying. Those will be your pieces of information with respect to where they are. Check in with them now and again. Ensure you hear is what is truly being said. Apply these aptitudes to yourself. You will be astonished at what you discover! Utilize these critical abilities to diminish the weight and stress that accompanies being an entrepreneur. Become that amazing guide for your customer!

Dr. Song S. Dweck was tested by her understudy to compose a book on the aftereffects of long periods of their exploration study. Dr. Song S. Dweck rose to the event and has composed this book, "Outlook: The New

Psychology of Success, and How we can Learn to Fulfill Our Potential" with the expectation that it will help the conventional individual comprehend that life is the thing that you make it and not what was managed to you during childbirth. She has written in basic language giving instances of conventional genuine individuals such as herself and her understudies, craftsmen like Picasso, sportsmen like Michael Jordan, the b-ball player and John McEnroe the tennis player, Marina Semyonova the incomparable Russian move teacher and CEOs of various organizations to give some examples. In the third section of her presentation she composes, "... you'll figure out how a basic conviction about yourself... guides an enormous piece of your life... Indeed it pervades all aspects of your life... " Thus she draws the peruser into the book, making the peruser one of her genuine models as the peruser gets oneself in these models.

Dr. Dweck presents the two kinds of mentalities, the fixed outlook and the development attitude in the principal segment of the book. She composes how she gained from multi year old children that disappointment could be transformed into a blessing in the event that you had the correct attitude. By giving them hard riddles to take a shot at, the children developed their scholarly abilities through exertion and didn't surrender. These children turned into her good examples in her quest for whether human characteristics are things that can be developed or are things bended in stone. Every individual has a one of a kind hereditary gift however understanding, preparing, and individual exertion take them the remainder of the way.

Dr. Dweck's twenty years of research has demonstrated that the view you receive for yourself significantly influences the manner in which you lead your life. She composes that, on the off chance that you accept that your characteristics and qualities are bended in stone and can't be changed then you have a fixed mentality. What's more, in the event that you accept that esteemed characteristics and qualities can be created and developed then you have a development outlook.

Fixed outlook individuals accept that a person's insight, quality and characteristics are a fixed amount which can't be expanded. On the off chance that they are doing great in school, at that point they are more brilliant than the other people who are not progressing admirably. In the event that they do well in games, at that point they have ability given them during childbirth. They invest energy to demonstrate that they are better in the characteristics managed to them just to demonstrate they were managed a sound portion and that they are not insufficient. On the off chance that something doesn't work for fixed attitude individuals they constantly accuse something different.

Development outlook individuals endeavor to improve consistently. They don't kick back and consider their to be as the last objective. In their brains there is consistently opportunity to get better. They have no opportunity to sit and consider themselves to be the best or superior to other people. They have no opportunity to sit and believe that they have an extraordinary ability. They are caught up with considering how they can improve it and what changes they can make if something expected went poorly. To them if something doesn't go right it's not disappointment it is a test to discover approaches to get it going.

In the second segment of the book, Dr.Dweck, takes us through her exploration voyage of fixed outlook and an adventure of development mentality through a few arrangements of eyes. Demonstrating how these two attitudes represent the deciding moment individuals in their day by day lives. In individual games she gives a case of John McEnroe fixed outlook in tennis. He was a splendid player who accepted on ability not exertion and buckling down. When he didn't win he accused something different. Like when he reprimanded the framework disliking the game any more. He would not assume liability. Micheal Jordan then again has a development outlook. On the off chance that he missed an objective he would proceed to rehearse for a few hours attempting to make sense of why he missed it In group activity the creator gives a case of Couch John Wooden who was strategically and deliberately normal however proceeded to win ten national titles. Mentor Wooden a development attitude, discloses to us he was great at getting players to fill jobs as a feature of a group. He thought about the sentiments of the players. Fixed outlook like Coach Bobby Knight picked players for ability. He was a fantastic mentor yet utilized the despot way to deal with win. The triumphant were brief and broke people's characters all the while.

In corporate organizations the creator uses General Electric CEO, Jack Welch, as the fixed attitude who figured out how to lower himself to a development outlook and as he developed in his mentality the organization developed simultaneously. Lee Iacocca whose fixed outlook is a great idea to bring the organization up to the top in a rush however then you have to dispose of him before he breaks it. Portage engine organization did only that and Lee Iacocca was unsettled. Fixed outlooks pioneers are progressively worried about being legends and put their self image before the welfare of the organization. The creator gives case of Enron as an organization that broke in the hands fixed mentality high echelon keen individuals. Enron utilized savvy individuals with ability and paid the greatest cost of shutting the organization. Enron is a genuine case of mindless obedience where administrators escape with their brightness and prevalence and settle on disastrous choices.

In affection, these two mentalities can represent the moment of truth a relationship. In her exploration, Dr. Dweck, discovered that fixed attitudes feel judged and marked by dismissal in a separation. They additionally picked retribution as a way to get at the individual who hurt them. Development attitudes pardoned, gain from it and proceed onward. The creator gives Hilary Clinton for instance who pardoned her better half and went to dropping so as to spare her relationship. Time and exertion is expected to develop the passionate aptitudes that are expected to keep a relationship.

Dr. Dweck, closes this third segment with the impact that guardians', instructors' and mentors' mentalities have on kids that are under their consideration. In her exploration she discovered that youngsters decipher the guardians expressions of help and consolation in a fixed mentality approach. This sets them up for disappointment. For instance, "... You discovered that so rapidly! You are so brilliant... " is deciphered as "... In the event that I don't pick up something rapidly, I'm not shrewd... " She clarifies that guardians, instructors and mentors should abstain from giving commendation that judges their insight or ability yet acclaim them for the work that they put in. She proceeds to state guardians, educators, and mentors need to give equivalent time and thoughtfulness regarding the youngsters paying little heed to their underlying aptitudes. The kids will thusly give all and bloom. The creator calls attention to, "... As guardians, educators, and mentors we are depended with people groups' lives. They are our obligation and our inheritance... "

In the fourth area of the book, Dr. Dweck, sets out on the most satisfying piece of her work, watching individuals change. Individuals are not cognizant or mindful of their convictions. Dr Aaron Beck, a therapist, found that he could show them how to function with and change these convictions. What's more, intellectual treatment, one of the best treatments at any point created, was conceived. Dr Dweck, utilized workshops to test the path individuals of fixed mentalities managed data they were getting. She found that they put a solid assessment on each snippet of data. Something great prompted an exceptionally solid positive mark and something awful prompted an extremely solid negative name. Individuals with development outlook are likewise always checking what's happening, however their interior monolog isn't tied in with making a decision about themselves or others. They are delicate to positive and negative data, however they are sensitive to it's suggestions for learning and productive activity. Dr. Dweck additionally had workshop for understudies. The workshops require a huge staff to convey the material. So the workshop material was put on intelligent PC modules. The educators direct their classes through the modules, and called it Braintology. These mentality workshops put understudies responsible for their mind.

It is intriguing to take note of how a straightforward trademark like an attitude influences basic leadership in a wide range of the populace. An understudy in kindergarten, a CEO in billion dollar organization, a specialist at work in an emergency clinic, a sportsman at training and on the court, a gourmet specialist at a top of the line inn, determination of move understudies and a game group. Undergrads drop classes or drop out of school due to having a fixed attitude. A development outlook encourages you figure out how to manage outrage, and manage generalizations in racial and sexual orientation separation. It's very captivating.

Most mentors engage in instructing for one

amazingly convincing and profitable reason - on the grounds that they need to have a beneficial outcome to the lives of others.

As a mentor, the degree to which you can satisfy that goal is dependent upon two variables. Right off the bat, your expertise and viability as a mentor; and furthermore, on the quantity of customers you can influence through the use of your administrations. The reason for this article is to concentrate on the subsequent factor.

During the time spent helping individuals, it's likewise feasible for mentors to build up a productive way of life for themselves en route. Indeed, these targets are totally complimentary.

Numerous agents, including mentors, neglect to perceive the significant moral job that advertising plays in their business. In doing so they build up a mentality that is foolish to themselves, their business, and their customers.

As a mentor, you are good to go. How

adequately you work your business is totally dependent upon you. There are massively effective mentors (as far as customer numbers, pay and training results), and mentors that are scarcely ready to engraving out a living. The contrast between these boundaries isn't their instructing competency, yet rather their attitude. You might be an unbelievably able mentor, yet except if you have individuals willing to utilize your administrations, your aptitudes are of practically zero worth.

So what outlook does it take to be a fruitful mentor?

An effective instructing attitude:

- Puts the necessities of prospects and customers first;

- Actively tries to help customers achieve their destinations;

- Is compassionate to the requirements of customers and prospects;

- Doesn't restrain the administration offered to customers, and

- Acts as a moral counselor.

It takes a Marketing Mindset to be a fruitful mentor.

We consistently know about mentors that vibe just as showcasing is 'driving' and 'untrustworthy.' They feel as if it's too 'salesy' and don't feel great with it. For those mentors, we will clarify why showcasing is both morally substantial and economically vital.

CHAPTER FOUR

Clinical leadership behavior

There is a gigantic (and developing) volume of individuals in the public eye that would profit by instructing administrations. We should call these individuals planned instructing customers, or prospects. These prospects have explicit objectives they'd like to accomplish, or difficulties they'd like to survive, with the end goal of driving a superior and all the more satisfying life.

As a mentor you have a specific obligation of consideration to help these individuals. You can just start to help them once they're using your administrations. Promoting is the connection between the prospects want and your capacity to help them satisfy their longing.

Showcasing just winds up unscrupulous in the situation that you are not ready to satisfy your advertising guarantee to your customer. In this occurrence you've misdirected your customer, either purposely or unwittingly, and have acted dishonestly.

On the reason that prospects will look for a mentor to help them achieve their particular objectives, it's the moral commitment of mentors to help prospects select a mentor that will best have the option to help them. To do this mentors ought to completely, extensively and straightforwardly reveal to prospects what administrations they offer; where their claims to fame lie; what experience they have; how they've helped individuals with comparative wants previously; and how utilizing their administrations will profit them. Or then again to state it all the more basically, to attempt advertising.

Financially Crucial

Showcasing is economically vital on the grounds that it connections prospects that longing a specific result with talented experts prepared to help them accomplish that result. It distinguishes you as somebody that might have the option to help prospects with their pre-qualified requirements. By searching out data on training administrations, prospects have officially distinguished for themselves:

1. That there are sure things throughout their life they'd like to accomplish or difficulties they'd like to survive.

2. That a mentor is an individual with the essential aptitudes and experience to help them.

3. That they are happy to put monetarily all the while.

The above is a critical point, and one that mentors need to acknowledge.

As we clarified before, mentors by and large originate from one of two ways of thinking as for showcasing.

The main way of thinking sees promoting to be 'driving' and 'salesy.' They originate from the worldview that by advertising you are proactively impacting somebody in their choices. Or then again explicitly that you may cause somebody to accomplish something they would not generally do. We call this line of reasoning the Influencing Paradigm.

The second way of thinking acknowledges that prospects are individuals that have distinguished for themselves their need to conjure change. Furthermore, they've distinguished that a mentor will help them roll out that improvement. They perceive that the prospect has made the scholarly interface between their needs and how they need those should be satisfied. We call this line of reasoning the Service Paradigm.

The manners of thinking of these two points of view are completely dipolar. One positions the prospect as somebody reluctantly impacted into using an administration, and different positions the prospect as a proactive individual equipped for deciding their needs that has effectively searched out instructing administrations.

As a mentor, it's important that you put yourself in the second worldview of reasoning. At exactly that point will you have the option to morally satisfy your goal of helping your customers. Furthermore, at exactly that point will you have the option to satisfy your harmonious objective of structure an effective training business.

By placing yourself in the Service Paradigm of idea you will perceive that to help customers meet their goals, you should:

- Actively advance your administrations through convincing promoting that obviously depicts what you can offer customers.

- Understand that as a mentor and a believed guide you are frequently in a superior situation of learning to discover your customer needs to help them accomplish their objectives.

- Be compassionate to the requirements of your customers and effectively offer answers for them through different items and administrations.

- Value your customer's astuteness and basic leadership capacity.

- Do not pre-empt your customer's needs and thus limit the range and extent of items and administrations you offer them.

- Always goes about as a moral consultant.

When you grasp the Service Paradigm to showcasing, you'll understand that promoting furnishes you with an a lot more prominent chance to satisfy your essential destinations - to help your customers, and to construct a fruitful training business. These goals become complimentary and you make a really win-win circumstance between the wants of your customers and your own wants.

In the second piece of this article we'll give you additional data on the best way to build up your Marketing Mindset and a Service Paradigm.

While an individual might want to improve a perspective or certain parts of their life so they can accomplish a particular objective, or set of objectives.

Simon Clarke has more than 15 years of experience as an essayist, business visionary and business authority. He is additionally the originator and Director of the Life Coaching Institute, Australia's driving mentor preparing association.

Despite the fact that training and initiative are interwoven and naturally connected, they are extraordinary and ought to be taken a gander at with an alternate focal point. As a mentor, you ought to comprehend the significance of being a pioneer when you are training, yet you ought to likewise perceive that instructing and administration are additionally isolated, particular characteristics and errands. This is particularly valid inside the structure of organizations.

How Coaching is Different from Leadership

Despite the fact that training and initiative cover from numerous points of view, instructing will in general be increasingly close to home and administration will in general be progressively broad and expansive. Initiative is tied in with recognizing and actualizing a dream for others to grasp and pursue. Training is tied in with helping other people distinguish objectives and make activity intends to arrive at those objectives.

A mentor and a pioneer frequently have similar results as a main priority yet regularly utilize diverse ranges of abilities to arrive at those results.

The Coaching Mindset

Training requires a confided regarding a customer or a worker. Mentors must be able to pose inquiries, to listen effectively, and to support customers or workers discover a way to self-acknowledgment and personal growth. With regards to an organization, mentors are frequently associated with day by day exercises, in the dirty subtleties of routine assignments and obligations. They should consistently build up some trust before endeavoring to discover results and arrangements. They work in association with the representatives to decide objectives and arrive at those distinguished objectives.

The Leadership Mindset

Pioneers normally have a fairly extraordinary

outlook and center than mentors. They should lead with a dream and rouse. They should get others to acknowledge their vision, make progress toward shared objectives, and accept what they accept. Like mentors, they should be great communicators. In contrast to mentors, they accomplish all the more telling and teaching. They should have the option to viably convey the purposes behind their vision; if the representatives don't comprehend the "why" they won't be completely put resources into the procedure and not as persuaded to arrive at the ideal results. Pioneers are making a superior future for the gathering; mentors are making a superior future each representative in turn.

Training and Leadership - Different however Equal

In spite of the fact that they are unique, initiative and instructing are both vital to the accomplishment of an organization. Training works more at the small scale level while initiative works all the more viably at the full scale level. Pioneers are progressively similar to designers and mentors are increasingly similar to manufacturers. A pioneer is increasingly similar to the lead trainer of a football crew, and a mentor is progressively similar to one of the organizers who work with explicit gatherings or positions.

A pioneer is at first worried about the 10,000 foot view however the subtleties additionally matter; a mentor is at first worried about the subtleties however the master plan likewise matters. The thing that matters is nearly as straightforward as: pioneers lead and mentors mentor!

Clinical nurse leader role

Numerous attendants with long stretches of nursing background behind them are moving in the direction of the following phase of their expert therapeutic vocations - as nursing teachers. Nursing instructors assume a basic job in the nursing calling, as they bring an abundance of real clinical experience to hold up under in their central goal to prepare the up and coming age of nurse attendants. In the event that you are a nurse attendant in the nightfall of your profession, or one who is simply searching for the following in a long queue of difficulties, a vocation as a nursing instructor might be only the change you need. It is unquestionably something that the remainder of the nation needs, as the approaching lack of qualified nurse caretakers might be considerably more serious than most specialists foresee because of a relating deficiency of qualified nursing teachers.

There are not many profession alternatives more compensating than that of a nursing teacher. There are not many in the business that have a greater amount of an effect on the psyches of new nurture than these instructors, as they can bestow attempted and tried nursing methods, yet their own one of a kind bits of knowledge into the delights and difficulties of life as a nurse attendant. For some nurse attendants who take up educating as another vocation, the chance to connect with their understudies in mentally testing activities once a day revives their very own enthusiasm for nursing and fight off the impacts of burnout.

You can discover nursing instructors at each degree of the instructive procedure, from undergrad concentrates to ace's projects. They serve the basic capacity of setting up each sort of nurse caretaker - from authorized down to earth attendants to future nurse caretaker instructors and industry pioneers. What's more, with that degree of duty there is an abnormal state of employer stability. The truth of the matter is that there are too few attendants in this nation, and excessively couple of instructors to teach the nurse caretakers we have to close the hole. That makes each nursing instructor's activity more secure, since the business would ill be able to stand to lose any of the educators it presently has.

Regardless of whether you are pondering a vocation in instructing, however need to work with patients also, there are open doors for you to seek after your interests. Indeed, there are many nurse attendant educators who figure out how to show nursing understudies the calling, while simultaneously giving nursing care to patients inside an emergency clinic or clinical setting. The capacity to keep in touch with patient consideration not just makes the change from nursing to showing simpler, yet additionally causes the teacher to stay aware of new methods and advancements as they are created.

On the off chance that you are hoping to make up your vocation in the medicinal services industry at that point being an attendant can generally be considered as perhaps the best choice in the present situation. Making a vocation as an attendant offers various advantages and rewards. Today, it won't not be right to state that on the off chance that you join the nursing field, you will join a profession that is one of the biggest in the field of social insurance in the United States. Truth be told, it is one of the most regarded occupations in America.

Causing a vocation in nursing to can really

give you a profound feeling of fulfillment as you could be one of only a handful couple of people who can be the pivotal connection among patients and specialists. Contingent on the circumstances, numerous patients invest unmistakably more energy collaborating with a nurse caretaker than they do with a specialist. Any doctors can analyze and simply endorse the meds or strategies to get fix from the sickness, however it is an attendant who really oversees the restoring method. Specialists may practice drug, however it is an attendant who performs and aides in appropriate time to time taking of medication.

It doesn't make a difference, regardless of whether you are going about as a Licensed Practical Nurse or a Registered Nurse, you might assume a significant job in making a genuine everyday contrast in the lives of countless patients and their families. You will be on the bleeding edges of the war on illness and damage, working fundamental life sparing innovation, checking patients or notwithstanding encouraging relatives. Past regard, there is likewise adaptability to pick where you wish to work, which clinic office you need to work or whether you need to work in an emergency clinic as low maintenance or full time.

These days the field of nursing in the United States is much of the time in necessity of very much prepared experts, which in the end demonstrates that by choosing a nursing vocation you will always have a work opportunity practically around the bend. The current circumstance of human services industry unmistakably demonstrates that the likelihood to fill the enormous number of open nursing occupations presently is low and troublesome. Truth be told, the vast majority of the urban communities in the United States are needing more nurse caretakers and the proportion is required to increment in next couple of years. According to the ongoing examination, as indicated by the U.S. Agency of Labor Statistics, around one million new and substitution nurse caretakers will be required by 2012, which unquestionably places enrolled nursing as the pioneer in occupation development. Adding to this, as indicated by American Hospital Association, nearly around 126,000 nurse attendants are as of now required to fill clinic work opening.

The issues identified with nursing include a careful assessment of nursing as hypothesis and practice. The job of the nurse caretaker expert particularly in regions of clinical basic leadership and the executives could be contemplated with regards to obstetrics and gynecological division or even crisis wards. The accentuation of most examinations is on intelligent work on utilizing Gibbs (1988) model of treatment and reflection. The need to pursue clinical rules as given by NICE or NHS have been underlined in a few examinations particularly featuring the significance of individual neatness and cleanliness in disease control.

The job of educated assent and clinical basic leadership if there should arise an occurrence of pregnancy with family ancestry of emotional wellness issues propose the focal job of the difficulties in the basic leadership process (Papers4you.com, 2006). The requirement for guiding and all encompassing consideration of patients have been stressed in clinical practice. The job of the attendant and the significance of appropriate information of clinical rules, NHS mandates and satisfactory medicinal preparing propose the urgent duty of the nurse attendant who assumes differed jobs from that of doctor to emergency clinic administrator. The investigations demonstrate the fluctuated ways to deal with nursing as if there should arise an occurrence of a discouraged patient, the accentuation is on guiding and mental help while in the event of treating a patient with hypertension or numerous wounds after mishap, intelligent practice on prompt measures pursued would be progressively significant, proposing an attention on patient focused results (Bowcutt, et al 2006).

Clinical administration is firmly identified with authority speculations and it is significant for the nurse caretaker to create sufficient initiative aptitudes to viably perform clinical obligations (Booth and Davies, 1991). The contrasts between the job of the wellbeing guest, nurse caretaker and birthing assistant as a rule practice have been considered. Social and human services arrangement and rules on clinical administration recommend a multidisciplinary synergistic working methodology for powerful clinical administration (Papers4you.com, 2006). Community oriented collaboration, all encompassing psychosocial treatment and appropriate designation of clinical assets are a portion of the issues that are significant inside escalated care units and for consideration of crisis patients. The moral and legitimate duties of an attendant expert and the restorative group all in all are generally guided by not simply clinical rules set by the Department of Health yet additionally by a group of devoted wellbeing experts inside the clinical setting.

The issues examined in the field of nursing incorporate clinical administration, collective collaboration, the job of the clinical nurse attendant specialist, the significance of intelligent practice, Gibbs (1988) Model, clinical administration and basic leadership, moral and legitimate issues in clinical consideration and comprehensive way to deal with treatment.

Pediatric clinical turn will set up a nursing understudy for giving medicinal consideration and instruction about maladies and treatment plans to youthful patients. Kids are not simply little grown-ups; their bodies work in various ways. The way that kids are as yet developing, the effect of the ailment or damage on their formative status must be considered. Also, in light of the fact that they are youthful, they might be progressively frightened or confounded by what is befalling them then what the result is. That is the reason they need pediatric nurse attendants who comprehend their specific needs.

Understudies should remember that youngsters have guardians and kin who are altogether included. Pediatric attendants work intimately with patient's families as a feature of the treatment procedure. One of the numerous things you may see yourself doing is imparting your nursing abilities to other. Your main responsibility is to give the kid's family the certainty and capacity to proceed with the minding job while at home. A pediatric nurse attendant will realize when to remain back and when to dominate if important when showing patient's and families certain abilities. It requires an uncommon arrangement of dispositions, tolerance and liberality to think about pediatric patients.

All nursing understudies are required to finish pediatric clinicals. Be that as it may, not all understudies are keen on thinking about pediatric patients and managing the families. This is an ideal opportunity to suck it up and overcome this pivot without a hitch. Despite the fact that you might not have any desire to be in this claim to fame after graduation, it will be a decent encounter and you will even now become familiar with a great deal. Prescriptions have a major influence in pediatric nursing, so figuring out how to ascertain pediatric measurements issues while in class is significant.

So as to get ready for clinicals you will in any case need everything that you use for grown-up wellbeing. Continuously convey dark ink pens, sharpie, pen light, recycled watch, and a stethoscope and a lot of persistence. The day preceding clinicals, your teacher will disclose to you what patient's you will have. Some of the time a friend in your gathering will be relegated as a group chief, they should drive to the nurse clinic the day preceding and get understanding data so as to dole out then to understudies. In the event that this is the circumstance, don't be reluctant to tell the group chief or your clinical educator that you might want to begin with a particular sort of patient. For instance, in the event that you are not happy with taking care of infants, you might need to demand a baby persistent first. That way, you can become acclimated to conveying and being around a tyke. For the most part when clinicals are over with, you will be certain enough to deal with an infant.

Pediatric clinicals for the most part involves doing a great deal of physical appraisals, perusing development graphs, giving intravascular meds and evolving diapers. There are a great deal of standards and guidelines that you should stick to, contingent upon the kind of office. Your talk classes ought to compare with what type illnesses and finding you will interact with at the nurse clinic. On the off chance that you appreciate working with infants and little children, you will feel right comfortable and have an incredible pediatric turn.

As referenced in the last issue, injury is an abrupt occasion that changes the course of an individual's life. The change can be transitory or perpetual and influences each part of being. All objectives and desires created over a lifetime are immediately stripped away with nothing to anticipate aside from agony and anguish. On the off chance that that weren't sufficient, the way to recuperation is full of obstructions, for example hurtful ways of dealing with stress and reactions, for example, streak backs, intermittent bad dreams, meddlesome contemplations, lack of sleep, constant torment, changes in self-perception, confidence and social connections, loss of autonomy, lower dissatisfaction resilience, fractiousness, unseemly alarm reactions to basic sounds and modifications in risk recognition. Furthermore, as referenced beforehand, the vast majority of us have encountered a horrendous accident at on schedule or another and every person experience different passionate reactions. In any case, given how the legitimate framework has advanced, it is presently vital to have the option to recognize resolvable reactions and responsive pathology. As needs be, we currently direct our concentration toward understanding the elements of how real specialists will recognize and resolve those reactions, with the goal that the lawyer can realize when there is authentic proof of pathology demonstrating an all-encompassing time of torment and enduring that meets lawful edge prerequisites.

Glimmer Backs

Among the majority of its astounding capacities the human mind is a faultless account gadget. All information improvements, for example, sound, light, shading, wind, warm changes, wetness, dryness, development, and so forth are recorded in the cerebrum's memory cells and stay for the length. The defectiveness of human memory is in the capacity to review. Regardless, everything that arrives at the mind through the five faculties gets recorded. In this manner, one of the issues with injury is that when there is a staggering abrupt contribution of boosts the cerebrum records it precisely as it happened with a bigger than-ordinary overlay. Thus, similarly as a plate as a point of confinement to how much data it will hold, the memory cell can just hold a limited measure of "information". So more cells are utilized to hold the memory of an occasion that produced more than the typical measure of boosts to which the individual was acclimated. Subsequently, the mind kicks into an "auto-replay" mode and remains there. This marvel is known as a "streak back".Accordingly, individuals who experience blaze backs depict remembering the occurrence again and again, with the recurrence and timing of the reiterations being eccentric. Along these lines this reaction for the most part shields the unfortunate casualty from having the option to do their standard exercises. Most patients that I have addressed said that it resembles being snared to an augmented experience PC and being stuck in a programming circle. This condition varies from having intermittent bad dreams in that by definition, it possibly happens when the patient is alert. Thusly, this injury reaction is aggravating and requires some instructing in how to deal with it. It most cases this characteristic marvel is self redressing of a short timeframe.

Intermittent bad dreams

Repeating bad dreams are a greater amount of a tricky issue than flashbacks since they are happening when we give up power over our bodies. Beside the numerous otherworldly and mental understandings of dreams, they are frequently a sign of musings and wants happening during the earlier day. This is the reason we frequently wind up getting things done in our fantasies that we could never consider accomplishing no doubt. By a similar token, the person in question, who as a rule has dreary considerations about various potential situations identified with the episode, will frequently remember the event, while envisioning, in manners that are much more awful than what really happened.On the other hand, the bad dream itself is of no result. The genuine issue is in how the individual reacts to it subsequent to awakening. A great many people wakeful from such scenes with an abnormal state of worry with expanded heart, respiratory rates, blood glucose levels and circulatory strain. There is some arrival of adrenalin and different hormones that should be activated just when there is threat. The typical enthusiastic reaction to the fantasy is feeling vexed and taking part in more contemplated the horrendous episode. Henceforth, the way to goals is discovering that such dreams must be dismissed as being of no significance and are a minor impression of what an individual was considering during the day. In this way, on the off chance that we buy in to this hypothesis as truth, we realize that decreasing the measure of time one spends contemplating the episode will lessen the recurrence and force of the bad dreams.

Over the top Thoughts

Over the top or meddling contemplations are the methods by which the unsafe passionate responses propagate. The manner of thinking offers ascend to the majority of the previously mentioned enthusiastic reactions for example outrage, uneasiness, melancholy, and so forth. In the division of the human condition (feeling versus keenness), the negative enthusiastic segment of the mind-body has equivalent access to the thinking mechanical assembly of the cerebrum. Henceforth contemplations regularly exude from this negative side. Moreover, negative emotions, for example, outrage, distress and uneasiness have a characteristic inclination to disperse similarly as bubbling water goes to steam and exhausts itself from the vessel. Hence, it requires an impressive exertion to propagate those destructive reactions. Also, as a feature of the normal human condition, there is a negative segment of each human that has a plan to achieve prompt delight at any expense and it doesn't have the ability to say something with the unintended outcomes. This "side" is ceaselessly at war with the astuteness which battles to keep up control in perspective on the undesirable outcomes of changing driving forces vigorously. Henceforth every choice is a response to the inquiry "Would it be a good idea for me to or shouldn't I?"

Accordingly, the adroit expert shows the customer to concentrate on great considerations. Which makes one wonder, "How is it conceivable to think just great contemplations with the majority of the hurt and anguish and with budgetary issues approaching seemingly within easy reach?" Although it is no simple undertaking, one can start by taking stock. Clearly, after an individual catastrophe, there are probably going to be some perpetual misfortunes. All in all, what is the most intelligent activity first? Consider the rest of the resources for see what there is to work with. The one clear thing that the vast majority ignore is, "I have endure. I am as yet alive." The survivor should be both glad and appreciative for that one certainty. This is a vital component, in light of the fact that there can be no advancement generally. The nearness or nonappearance of this dynamic in any treatment session coming full circle in a specialist's report is a decent test for getting rid of malingerers.

Lack of sleep is a reaction to a progression of reactions. Agony, uneasiness, misery and anguish to give some examples are largely contributory to burglarizing an individual of their rest. We as a whole need a specific measure of normal sleep to work when things are going admirably. It turns out to be significantly progressively significant when one is recuperating from injury. The absence of rest meddles with mending on each level. In this manner, the way to recuperation must start with getting tranquil rest notwithstanding the majority of the elements that foil it. This leaves the unfortunate casualty in a predicament since the majority of the mind-body reactions that avert rest are heightened by the absence of it.Therefore, proficient assistance is required much of the time, notwithstanding when the physical wounds are generally minor. Nonetheless, most going to doctors will turn to recommending drugs that instigate rest and the patient gets practically zero opportunity to verbalize. The present arrangement of medicinal consideration doesn't permit much time for verbal connection with wellbeing experts. Indeed, even nurture, who are explicitly instructed for diagnosing and treating post awful reactions infrequently have opportunity to give helpful guiding in institutional settings. Along these lines, most hospitalized injury exploited people don't approach suitable treatment for antagonistic rest denying reactions during the early piece of their recovery.Consequently, it is left to relatives, huge others as well as private advisors to give a steady domain. This requires investing the energy expected to enable the patient to share their worries and grievances. Despite the fact that there are a couple of medication free procedures for initiating rest, for example, biofeedback, loosening up sounds and alleviating music, the best unwinding inducer is a consoling voice.

Modifications in Self Image (Body Image and Self Esteem)

Modifications in self-perception and confidence are visit reactions to injury. The shared factor is the means by which an individual characterizes their personality with respect to physical depiction, persona, gaining limit and job. We burn through the majority of our lives developing this open picture and afterward setting up barriers to ensure it. In perspective on that, injury tears away all strongholds and the individual is disregarded inclination helpless and. Accordingly, it resembles "The individual that I know to be me has quite recently disappeared and the beat up, powerless one lying in this bed is an all out outsider!"

To look at this loss of self all the more intently, the above situation makes one wonder, "For what reason does our own character idea that we buckled down to create throughout the years dissipate so effectively? One little shock and poof! gone." The appropriate response is that the mental self portrait isn't reality. It is only a dream emerging out of either an exact view of criticism from others, self-duplicity or a blend of both. So it ought to be nothing unexpected that at the time of a life changing occasion, the individual we recollected ourselves to be is gone. We are presently managing someone unique. Ok, yet it is in actuality such a stun, that it takes months or years to acclimate to the change. This is so on the grounds that we as a whole neglect to recall two essential standards of life: first, we have no power over the conditions of our being; and second, we overlook that, similar to the costs of gas and carrier tickets, life subject to change without notice.Accordingly, the customer needed to come to comprehend that mindfulness is unimportant recognition. Consequently, notwithstanding when injury happens causing perpetual damage there is no genuine modification or loss of self at its center. There is just an apparent change in the physical sign in light of the horrendous effect. Along these lines, since the quintessential individual is otherworldly fundamentally, a wrecked mirror changes the reflection, however the reflected item stays sound. This idea is the foundation of understanding the differentiation among debilitation and incapacity.

Modifications in social connections

Every individual is a connect to a few networks, for example, family, work, school, social club, athletic group, political affiliations, and place of love, and so on. We assume a job in every one of these gatherings, for example, part, pioneer, tyke, parent, life partner, specialist, chief, companion, etc. At the point when an individual winds up wiped out or harmed, the individual in question can't satisfy the jobs that had been built up and the connections change. Generally it means some type of job inversion between relatives. The individual upon whom others depended is currently needy upon them.Consequently, there are various enthusiastic reactions emerging out of unfulfilled desires, for example dissatisfaction, outrage, hatred and such. Albeit a few people meet people's high expectations and are glad to give the additional administrations expected to think about a friend or family member, regularly connections between relatives fall apart because of the passionate reactions of the injury understanding. The standard grievance from the companion or other relative is that the harmed individual ended up fractious, dreadful and now and then verbally oppressive. The weakening of the family connections is a result of intrinsic dangerous conduct driving forces that exists in potentia all people. These issues emerge on the grounds that the harmed individual in such cases shows the qualities of an egotistical obtuse animal who needs to control others. This is what number of individuals managing trepidation and anxiety.Therefore, the injury persistent who has exploited their relatives must utilize a differentiation called "assuming liability". This is a troublesome idea to take hold of on the grounds that the idea of the "debilitated job" is to be exonerated of responsibility. In this way the verbally mishandled relative takes the tongue lashing and attempts to stay unemotional until the individual loses it, strikes back and eventually leaves persuaded of the requirement for self safeguarding.

Attack of Privacy and Loss of Independence

Being harmed consistently brings about two noteworthy changes: Invasion of Privacy and loss of freedom. My first teacher in the nursing program that I went to stated, "To figure out how to be a decent nurture you should initially realize what it resembles to be a patient." Thus our first exercise was about intrusion of protection and shame. The fundamental features were that private capacities and body parts were in plain view. In a showing emergency clinic, during terrific rounds, the going to doctors go with a gathering of eight or ten assistants and inhabitants (doctors in-preparing) to see each alloted understanding. Each specialist leads a physical assessment before their associates and educator and explains the discoveries and treatment plan. I have had numerous customers grumble that it resembled being in plain view in Macy's window.Although this situation has its avocations, it can't be translated as something besides an attack of security. The hospitalized individual needs to surrender their requirement for unobtrusiveness and endure open revealing so as to determine the helpful advantages of conclusion and treatment. Be that as it may, too intentioned as it might be, the abrupt revealing of ones body within the sight of a few eyewitnesses causes mortification and shame, which thusly brings about expanded pressure and retards recuperating. This issue likewise strikes a lesser degree in the doctorã¢â'¬â"¢s office and in the home.On the other hand, while the onus is on experts and other guardians to stay delicate to an individual's requirement for nobility, numerous individuals can obstruct the pressure initiating shame reaction. They basically settle on a choice to acknowledge that in a therapeutic setting individuals have just a clinical intrigue and that the activities are altogether planned to profit the patient. Truth be told, any shyness displayed in such a setting would be a bogus humility in light of the fact that the individual would act against their very own interest.Regarding the loss of freedom, this is firmly connected to the attack of security issues in light of the fact that harmed individuals need to depend on parental figures to perform private capacities like utilizing the latrine. The individual more often than not needs to do this at the bedside and hang tight for another person to divert it and give individual cleanliness. Acclimating to this is to a greater extent an issue on the grounds that, notwithstanding when the humiliation issues have been settled, there more often than not stays a solid disdain against relying upon others for things that we regularly manage without idea. What troubles some is the loss of control and others harbor a dread of turning into a burden. One compelling way that advisors help their customers adapt to this quandary is for the reliant individual to discover that the individual in question is making a commitment to the parental figure's prosperity. Individuals need to feel required. The reliance of someone else inspires the statement of adoration and imparts a feeling of direction. In this manner, when one individual has a need that is satisfied by another the beneficiary is really making a bigger commitment than the provider. Given this qualification, the needy individual can figure out how to acknowledge the administrations with a feeling of euphoria and appreciation.

CHAPTER FIVE

The contemporary leadership theory

Disappointment resistance relates to the time allotment that an individual is eager to hang tight for the satisfaction of needs and needs before having a fit. Despite the reasons, the genuine conduct seems like the influenced individual has a permit to be awful mannered and contentious. It can likewise be portrayed as backward and tyke like. Moreover, there is a large group of negative results in making harm others and destroying connections as recently referenced. This can be very costly.Another terrible the truth is that injury doesn't make another individual. It simply strips away the exterior and permits the subsurface very much controlled offensive attributes to show in the mind-body. The harmed individual with low disappointment resistance ends up shouting at the individuals who are doing their best to give administration. Despite the fact that this is unwanted conduct, as a rule it isn't the typical lead of the person in question and hence there is a method for bringing the creature back leveled out.

Touchiness

In spite of the fact that there is some cover among crabbiness and low dissatisfaction resilience, the previous doesn't really include giving oneself consent to be hostile. This manifestation talks more to the way the mind-body react to upgrades, for example, light and sound. The spirit, which is a profound substance, associates with the physical world through the mind-body. At the point when an individual winds up bad tempered because of injury or other wellspring of mind-body changes, the instrument for response to boosts is in overdrive.For model, when we are alert and approaching our ordinary exercises, discussions occurring in typical tones don't ordinarily cause an issue. Be that as it may, in the event that you need to tune in to a similar discussion while you are attempting to rest, that is an alternate story. You will blow up and wind up telling the culprits, "shut up!" The bad tempered individual responds to ordinary discussions and different sounds similarly constantly. By and by, by and large it is a brief circumstance eased by a calm domain.

Immediate Conditioned Reflexes

To comprehend the idea of the immediate molded reflexes and how to determine them, we need comprehend the differentiation that in light of boosts, there are two sorts of activity; that which is thought subordinate and that which is not.For the mind-body, each improvement summons a reaction that outcomes in a change. In this way, the spirit's activity can be modified. For example, if your vehicle hits a pothole that thumps the front wheels askew, your directing will be influenced in light of the fact that you should alter the vehicle's new propensity to veer off to one side or right. Going further, if nothing happens other than the expansion of a memory, that by itself comprises a perpetual change. Consequently, the otherworldly pith, which is worried to keep its vessel on course to complete its central goal, will settle on a choice whether to utilize the idea, discourse and additionally activity to respond.However, there is likewise the reflex bend which is the capacity to react to improvements without earlier idea. This is the place the body has figured out how to respond a specific method to limit damage. The nerve motivation never arrives at the mind on the grounds that there is a prearranged reaction good to go the minute the drive arrives at the spinal rope. The reflex curve is a device for protection. It capacities at the essential creature level since it is there only for self-protection.

This idea relates to the capacity to rapidly pull back the hand from a hot article without contemplating it first. Subsequently, this talk is focused on the unexpected modification of the majority of the educated reactions to boosts created over a lifetime by want, learning and framing propensities. Similarly as with some other existing or potential nurse issue, the goals for fixing the unexpected change forced by injury lies in how the connection between the soul and the mind-body was influenced.

Wrong Startle Responses

Wrong surprise reactions are a genuine wellbeing danger since they cause unnecessary measures of pressure. Being surprised is a distinct response to an unforeseen event. There is an unexpected arrival of adrenalin with an expansion in pulse and circulatory strain. With this condition the trigger can be any ecological sound or sight that would some way or another not deliver any impact, for example, shutting an entryway, closing a kitchen cupboard or dropping the latrine situate. The reason for this isn't well understood.However, the nature of injury is to such an extent that it generally occurs all of a sudden and there is typically a specific sound or sight related with it like road clamor or the sound of the accident. In this vein, the mind-body learns right now of effect to connect any abrupt surprising boosts with inalienable danger.Moreover, during typical action we can get a great deal of contribution through our five faculties without being overpowered. Consequently we can hold our very own recognizable method for being or try to embrace diverse responsive practices. Notwithstanding, during an awful accident we are besieged with heightened upgrades that establish a long term connection, similar to a meteor that pummels into the earth making a cavity that is a lot bigger in measurement than the grandiose missile.The goals is genuinely basic. The unfortunate casualty needs to re-figure out how to react to different destinations and sounds. One successful technique is to have relatives more than once make clamors in the house while making certain the harmed individual knows about when it will occur. One woman that I advised, who was "seizing each clamor" understood that she just drew back from unforeseen sounds. Along these lines, at my proposal, she got her better half and youngsters to advise her before they made their typical clamors. Following half a month she progressed toward becoming re-acquainted with the different family unit rattles and was never again being frightened.

Improper Fight or Flight Responses

The way toward creating "learned" autonomic reactions is one of memory. The cerebrum "recalls" the improvement and records a "modified" reaction. This makes the individual go energetically without earlier idea at whatever point that specific trigger shows up once more. These "stress activators" can be any site, sound, contact, smell or sort of "feel" that bears a comparability to the harmful occasion. Thus the unfortunate casualty sees threat and the mind-body reacts in like manner with an adrenalin surge that produces fast heart beat and breaths, raised circulatory strain and extraordinary enthusiastic fervor which can bring about a fit of anxiety. Regularly the risk isn't genuine and if this condition sustains it can turn into a crazy delusion.In different cases, I have treated individuals who were startled of heading to the degree that they imagined that they were going to bite the dust while the vehicle was still in the garage. Also, there was a woman mail bearer who had been destroyed by a German shepherd and was scared of canines and the structure examiner harmed by a detonating evaporator who was petrified of turning on his stove or broiler. These responses were all the aftereffect of quick molded reflex. The injury delivered such a mind-boggling impression in the memory cells of the cerebrum, which "instructed" the mind-body that the episode would happen again any second. the mail bearer accepted that each pooch was an awful man eater; and the structure overseer was persuaded that any warmth delivering apparatus was going to explode.Therefore, the arrangement is to learn not to be terrified of those triggers, for example, a vehicle, a canine, or a stove. Despite the fact that the goals might be straightforward it is difficult. Figuring out how to dispose of these injury incited condition reflexes is a dull errand yet should be cultivated or the unfortunate casualty's personal satisfaction will be for all time and seriously impaired.First, since we are animals of propensity, the mind picks up quality by reiteration. On the off chance that you articulate something regularly enough you will begin to trust it. Subsequently, the unfortunate casualties need to more than once state so anyone can hear that there is nothing to fear and that it was just a solitary demonstration of the Almighty (some would want to consider it a "crack accident").Second, the individual who is terrified to drive a vehicle needs to go vigorously and get in the driver's seat. Be that as it may, this must be a bit by bit process. The unfortunate casualty ought not begin pushing immediately. There is a radio television show character in

South Florida by the name of JoyceKaufman who as of late turned out to be seriously harmed in a cruiser mishap. She called it "a life changing occasion" and was pondering whether she ought to ever get back on her cruiser again. When she returned broadcasting live, numerous audience members brought in saying that an individual frightened of driving after a mishap ought to get into the vehicle and start driving quickly to beat the dread. That would be a horrendous mix-up in light of the fact that an individual who is anxious and unsteady would be a threat to self as well as other people out and about. The individual must do this bit by bit and reconstruct some self-assurance. It must resemble figuring out how to drive all over again.Finally, on account of the destroying injured individual, figuring out how to be agreeable around mutts again is progressively dangerous, yet can be practiced. For this, one would need constrained presentation to an accommodating creature. I would pick an old pooch that can't do anything other than lie around throughout the day. Despite the fact that this individual may never turn into a pooch darling, the unfortunate casualty should have the option to stroll down the road without being threatened within the sight of other individuals' mutts. Any released bizarre creature ought to be reason to worry, yet the previous chomp unfortunate casualty can build up some solace level within the sight of pooches secured behind a fence or hung on a rope.

A culture of safety

There are various meanings of culture. Everybody appears to have their own interpretation of it. In the wake of working with more than 85 medicinal services associations in the previous 8 years to enable them to make and continue a culture of wellbeing dependent on the prescribed procedures of high dependability associations, I have come to accept:

The core of this definition is the thing that individuals do at the day by day snapshots of truth. Inherently, you realize what a critical point in time is - the tens, if not hundreds, of little choice focuses each social insurance expert experiences throughout their day by day exercises. A choice point is the place a decision must be made. You can do "An" or "B." You can accomplish something, or nothing. You can say something, or state nothing. You can do it the correct way, or utilize a work-around. You can do it carefully, or negligently. Huge numbers of these choices are chosen nearly on the intuitive level, some of the time habitually - without monitoring choosing.

Changing society starts with changing how people think right now of truth. On the off chance that you can change how they think, influence why they do what they do - at that point you can change how they act right now of truth. On the off chance that we can change their reasoning long enough to influence how they follow up on a monotonous premise, at that point we can enable them to create propensities. Propensities are those moves we make nearly without speculation - it's simply the way we "work together" on an individual level. Changing propensities changes our character. Character is our main thing, again nearly at the subliminal level, particularly when we think nobody is viewing or nobody will know.

Eventually, culture is controlled by the aggregate character of the majority of the individuals in the association. Their character is controlled by their propensities. Their propensities are controlled by how they more than once act at snapshots of truth. Their activities right then and there are controlled by how their manners of thinking have been affected. So on the off chance that you need to change culture, you should change character, and in the event that you need to change character you should change propensities, and on the off chance that you need to change propensities you should change redundant activities, and on the off chance that you need to change activities you should change how individuals think.

As far as I can tell the best method to change how individuals believe is through administration activities. These activities incorporate advances like:

Over-imparting what must be done, how it

must be done, and why it must be finished;

Adjusting the majority of the records that portray how business is done in the association with the way of thinking of how it ought to be finished;

Open and monotonous affirmation and compensating of the ideal activities at the snapshots of truth;

Steady training for those requiring improvement and willing to improve;

Forcing negative ramifications for those reluctant to change how they think and act.

To change how individuals act right now of truth, preparing is best. "Telling" isn't preparing. Incredible preparing that changes activities is experiential, between disciplinary, contextual investigation based, takes into account practice, and offers continuous criticism and fortification on execution. Successful preparing gives both the individual and the group a chance to rehearse the activities required in a learning domain so they will skillfully be utilized right now of truth.

To guarantee those activities are over and again utilized when required and along these lines made into a propensity, designed apparatuses are best. Apparatuses like agendas, conventions, correspondence contents, institutionalized interchanges, and instructions aides help individuals utilize the correct activity at the correct minute. The apparatuses fill in as a compelling capacity; if the device is utilized accurately as a major aspect of the predictable every day work process, the individual must choose the option to make the correct move over and again and in this manner builds up a successful propensity.

Gradually, minute by minute, individual by individual, propensities are instilled and character changes. As character changes, the way of life likewise changes. The magnificence of the LifeWings philosophy is that every one of the parts important to influence thinking, activities, and propensities are worked in to our procedure and our master facilitators and mentors show and instruct the aptitudes to pursue the way of life evolving recipe.

Improving the future scene of our nation's social insurance framework relies on making and supporting societies where medicinal services experts are permitted to be prepared to do all they were made to be.

How about we start the dialog by asking some extreme, presumably insolent, questions.

Does your association genuinely energize a Culture of Safety?

Does your Culture of Safety really start at the highest point of your association, and do your pioneers (possibly you?) in reality live and exhibit that culture each working day?

Are your laborers accused (or feel they may be accused) in the event that anything turns out badly?

Are your Health and Safety frameworks also characterized and executed as (state) your bookkeeping frameworks, or other line-of-business frameworks?

See - we let you know these may be intense inquiries.

This article is about the idea of utilizing programming as a method for supporting your Health and Safety forms. Be that as it may, how about we not affront your knowledge by saying 'simply use programming to change your way of life'.

Programming can positively help you to empower a culture of wellbeing, and in doing so will decrease hazard presentation to your executives and standards by exhibiting your duty to this culture. We should accept for the minute that you were to introduce Health and Safety programming; in what capacity may that move you towards your objective of changing your way of life?

Right off the bat it's tied in with empowering the entire group to carry Health and Safety to the 'cutting edge'. For most hazard inclined organizations, this bound to be the shop floor, the processing plant floor, the structure site or the cowshed. Unquestionably not simply the 'workplace'. In any case, most wellbeing and security frameworks (especially the assortment that sit in a folio on a residue secured rack) are worked by back-office staff.

Imagine a scenario in which Health and Safety was everybody's duty, especially the individuals who need to play out their activity in the very condition that compromises them and their partners.

In a perfect world you'd take a gander at a cloud-based arrangement as it doesn't require establishment of programming onto the PC, tablet or cell phone. By utilizing normal 'program' innovation, it's conceivable to sidestep the workplace and get directly to the area of perils. With programming running on these kinds of gadgets, your clients can rapidly begin to take responsibility for detailing and Toolbox and Tailgate sessions.

Site-Specific Safety Plans

Take the case of Site-Specific Safety Plans or SSSPs. These comprise of a heap of reports including Explanatory Notes, Checklists, Hazard Registers, Notifications of Hazardous work, Task Analysis worksheets, and Evacuation and Emergency plans. Each Plan must be created in explicit detail, for every individual site that you're presently chipping away at.

For most associations, these can mean a gigantic regulatory overhead and along these lines the undertaking is generally assigned to authoritative staff. Frequently, the main way this can work is for them to deliver different photocopied adaptations of nonexclusive reports.

Yet, utilizing programming, the site Supervisor can redo the Plan on their tablet, produce a solitary record group containing upwards of 20 individual archives, press the print catch, and out it flies on paper or as a PDF. Notwithstanding, this time it's been created by a topic master. At work. With authorized data.

Dangers

We should take Hazard Registers as another case of specialist possession. Envision the comfort of having the option to finish a Hazard report on your cell phone, and after that snap a picture on the gadget and transfer it as a major aspect of the Hazard Register.

Perils can be evaluated on an ISO-31000 agreeable hazard framework. Put just, fairly attempting to control every one of your risks on the double, this enables you to concentrate on those with the most potential for issue. Also, you can continue bringing down the 'satisfactory hazard' edge; thus delivering a more secure working environment.

The complexity between office laborers and every other person

For certain associations, the hole between the individuals who 'drive a work area' and the individuals who work 'on the devices' is more than physical. A few specialists discover it truly baffling that their working practices seem, by all accounts, to be being controlled (in any event in a wellbeing and security sense) by partners who have never worked in a dangerous situation.

Envision how freeing it tends to be for versatile or open air laborers to feel drew in with a genuinely useful Health and Safety framework, and not only one which sits on an office rack some place. The expanding utilization of hand-held gadgets is presently freeing them, and enabling them to assume liability for their very own procedures.

Relieving hazard for Directors

Chiefs need to show that they have found a way to protect their laborers. That they have drawn in their staff in the way of life of wellbeing. That they have done their best, and still the individual has accomplished something idiotic or careless or unapproved or unfortunate.

Will a functioning Health and Safety framework spare a heavy fine or even a correctional facility term? We can't state. Be that as it may, we can say that it can bring down the hazard that you'll be the substitute in case of a fiasco. Considerably more critically, we can say that there is probably going to be a lower danger of the debacle occurring in any case.

Presentation:

Wellbeing in the working environment is experiencing change: advancing from a discretionary extra to a consistence need, firms are presently progressively perceiving the numerous advantages of creating, and focusing on, a solid security culture. These range from expanded staff assurance and expanded profitability, to decreased damage related costs, aggressive protection premiums and improved turnover benefits and notoriety.

Nonetheless, promising a culture of security includes more than unimportant lip administration. Wellbeing orientated qualities, long haul responsibilities to firm-wide security, and reliable solid activities will figure out which associations will receive the benefits of making and keeping up a powerful wellbeing society.

What is implied by a "Wellbeing Culture", and for what reason is it significant?

Security in the working environment spares lives; it likewise sets aside cash. As per the 2013 Liberty Mutual Workplace Safety Index, US organizations lose in excess of a billion dollars per week in pay expenses emerging from the 10 most regular working environment wounds and diseases - occurrences which could be averted with legitimate security measures set up. These figures don't represent the related profitability misfortunes and authoritative costs, which are evaluated to add up to a further $120 billion, yearly.

The standards held should be appropriately and reliably conveyed to staff. The words utilized, just as the tone, will put forth for all faculty how truly the board takes security in the working environment. Staff individuals will consistently submit their general direction to the administrative correspondence they get, obvious or something else; if these are reliably positive and strong, the establishments of a positive wellbeing society will be laid.

Similarly as with any circumstance, be that as it may, activities talk more intense at that point words. Any activities, anyway little, which chiefs or supervisors take to empower, advance or bolster wellbeing in the work environment will have a constructive thump on impact on all faculty. (As a conclusion, positive verbal correspondence will have little sway on the off chance that it isn't supported up by comparatively positive activities.) The best activities which ranking staff individuals can take are those which unmistakably remunerate security arranged conduct in others. This, more than anything, will communicate something specific of the significance of security to the association.

By and large, an association's wellbeing society is a blend of its qualities, correspondences and, most importantly, its activities.

Building up your Firm's Safety Culture

All organizations have a wellbeing society - in any case, not all have a positive one. Before you can find a way to build up your organizations, you have to figure out what kind of wellbeing society is as of now set up.

Distinguish Your Own Culture

The initial step is to speak with the faculty entrusted with the association's wellbeing - the suitable administrator or specialist. This will give input on what the firm would in a perfect world want its qualities to be. The truth, nonetheless, might be very extraordinary, and must be surveyed starting from the earliest stage: by speaking with all staff individuals, and distinguishing their impression of the association's wellbeing society.

One of the most proficient and thorough methods for speaking with a staff about its wellbeing society is to create and flow polls. To guarantee genuineness and openness, any such poll ought to be expressed to be without unknown from negative results, and be meaning to act emphatically on the data accumulated.

What's more, a poll should address an expansive scope of wellbeing society markers; as a guide, one of the pioneers in Safety Culture, Dan Petersen, distinguished 20 security the executives classifications, including: Attitude Towards Safety, Inspections, Employee Training, Supervisor Training, Involvement of Employees, and Operating Procedures. Such classifications merit considering as a guide when creating or inspecting surveys.

Having decided how solid - or something

else - your association's wellbeing society is, you would then be able to assess the situation and structure an arrangement for pushing forward. On the off chance that your firm has a frail culture, at that point the initial steps to take are to liaise with senior administration to distinguish the company's arrangement. As a security official, you may at first be met with obstruction, more often than not in connection to the apparent expense of execution. A portion of the expenses and impacts of an inability to build up a solid wellbeing society have been set out above, and ought to be imparted as important.

Create and Improve Your Firm's Culture

Independent of your association's current situation, there are various advances that can be taken to improve a company's way of life. Clearly, all move made ought to think about the association's business, size and structure, yet here are a few instances of activities which can apply independent of such limits:

• Involve Your Staff

The most ideal approach to build up a solid wellbeing society is to include all work force. Engaging staff sends the message that their job in the accomplishment of the firm is significant, and assumes a significant job in empowering staff assurance and pride. Staff can be associated with a heap of ways, from giving criticism on firm strategies, having a wellbeing contact official, making a security panel, or creating plans appropriate to explicit offices.

• Operate starting from the top

The most ideal approach to guarantee safe conduct in the work spot is to have it reflected from the board. Any wellbeing strategy executed should be shown by senior administration and leaders.

• Introduce a Mentor Program

A security guide program is a compelling method for acquainting new staff individuals with the wellbeing society. Just as making inspirational desires from existing laborers, it makes good examples for approaching staff to pursue.

• Implement Effective Training

Preparing itself isn't adequate: it must be compelling. To this end it ought to be:

Complete enough - a lot of data one after another is bound to be overlooked;

Progressing - one-off preparing isn't sufficient. To show a genuine responsibility to wellbeing, preparing should be customary and occasional;

Adaptable - powerful preparing ought to have the option to oblige all degrees of crowd;

Applicable - tailor each instructional meeting as indicated by the fitting division; and

Natural - it should "develop" with the staff

individuals.

• Diarise Safety Reviews

To be completely viable, a security program should likewise consolidate standard audits. It is worth, thusly, thinking about intermittent gatherings to examine and survey wellbeing, looking at inner issues and occurrences, yet in addition to talk about any applicable issues which have happened inside the business which could affect security in your firm.

• Display Your Safety Message

Perceivability is key in making a culture. Publicizing your qualities tells your staff that you are not kidding about, and focused on, your wellbeing society.

• Recognize and Encourage Positive Action

Methods for doing this incorporate making an occasional Safety Worker grant, publicizing positive wellbeing activities over the firm or even the business, or actualizing littler, less formal intends to feature inside the association steps taken by people.

• Communicate Effectively

At long last, it isn't sufficient for an association's administration to convey its qualities and thoughts; powerful correspondence should be a two-way occasion. To guarantee a solid wellbeing society, an association must tune in to its staff, and make the channels for successful two-way correspondence. Wellbeing requires the contribution everything being equal, and a security culture should unequivocally grasp and incorporate all individuals from the association.

The Role of Safety Management Systems

Security Management Systems are, deservedly, expanding in prominence, as associations perceive that wellbeing in the working environment isn't just a consistence issue, yet additionally a matter of powerful hazard the executives.

At the point when hitched with positive security based qualities, powerful correspondence and dynamic activities, a SMS is a basic wellbeing instrument, major for estimating wellbeing, and evaluating the association's improvement. It empowers staff individuals to rapidly and effectively convey approaches and activities, and to execute and accomplish security objectives. Besides, an expansive framework will feature wellbeing perils and dangers, encouraging deterrent measures, and supporting danger the board.

Moreover, the usage of a SMS is a solid methods for an association to exhibit the two its interest in, and pledge to, a positive, solid security culture.

CHAPTER SIX

Appreciating others

No curve balls here, the most recent study by Reuters and the University of Michigan expressed, "U.S. buyer certainty melted away in late July to its least ebb since April on developing negativity about the long haul monetary standpoint, particularly about pay and occupations, a review appeared on Friday, even as certain financial analysts figure the longest subsidence in decades might ease." Guess what, most shoppers are additionally representatives or they are identified with somebody who is delegated a worker. So a sensible presumption a pioneer can make is that your representatives are likewise not extremely hopeful, and regularly cynicism influences spirit and execution contrarily.

I likewise find that pioneers are in the doldrums and are thinking that its hard to be certain and battle to keep their very own spirit up, don't worry about it keeping their representatives' confidence up.

The activity is made additionally testing in light of the fact that the typical assurance promoters have been cut and decreased, making it a test to give workers a lift and to tell them that they are basic to overcoming this subsidence.

Well it's not as depressing as you and they may think! There is an integral asset that pioneers, guardians and life partners can use to slice through the negativity, fortify connections and influence assurance and execution in a positive manner.

I call it Active Appreciation. This article centers around an apparatus and expertise that when connected legitimately will support confidence and improve execution and it could possibly enable you to feel not so much pushed but rather more idealistic.

Dynamic Appreciation is an amazing asset that when genuinely conveyed by pioneers, it will expand commitment, propel change and improve confidence. So for what reason don't pioneers use it all the more frequently? What they normally let me know is, "I thought about it however I didn't have opportunity." and "I thought about it, yet before I could tell the individual I became involved with something different and overlooked." I've additionally heard, "I'm not here to make individuals feel better; they ought to acknowledge they have occupation." And, "I have a business to run; if individuals need embraces, their working for an inappropriate organization." Although, I can comprehend the reasons of insufficient time and overlooking, and contemplates unequivocally propose that the last dispositions smother, if not kill abnormal state commitment and execution, both present lost chances to accomplish what they need - a spurred, drew in and submitted workforce. Furthermore, in the present recessionary and violent business atmosphere when more is being removed, Active Appreciation is a blessing, that has least cost, yet is exceptionally esteemed by workers and has a high ROI.

As of late I requested a display of approval from a gathering of 50 representatives to the accompanying inquiry. What might you esteem more from your manager, an occasion gathering or regular expressions of appreciation? Expressions of gratefulness were the definitive victor. Pioneers disparage that they are so imperative to the individuals who work for them and how amazing their expressions of gratefulness can be in structure and fortifying connections and execution. Being perceived and acknowledged, especially by somebody who has the status of a pioneer, educator or parent, is an essential human want. Neglected, it can strain connections - leaving individuals feeling undesirable and overlooked.

The Gallup Organization in studying in excess of 15 million workers found that commitment and execution is made, fortified and supported when pioneers energize representative advancement, exhibit their minding and give workers acknowledgment at regular intervals. Dynamic Appreciation incorporates every one of these variables.

It's likewise intriguing to take note of that when I request that pioneers ponder somebody in their life who had or positively affects their vocation and life, and what did these people do to accomplish this status in their life, they constantly distinguish social and enthusiastic factors, for example, He regarded my feeling, he thought about me, she gave me legitimate input, she supported me. These individual reflections bolster what numerous examinations have distinguished: the intensity of acknowledgment and gratefulness is an incredible asset in structure and fortifying connections, commitment and execution.

There will in general be a hole in observation among pioneers and workers with respect to thankfulness and acknowledgment. Pioneers will in general react with a reverberating yes when posed the inquiry, "Do you welcome the individuals who work for you?" When I chat with representatives and ask them, "Do you feel increased in value?", the reactions are blended, best case scenario. This hole is the thing that I call the "gratefulness hole". It doesn't make a difference, as pioneer, in the event that you think you value your representatives - what makes a difference is if your workers feel increased in value. Shutting this hole can have a huge effect in the degree of commitment and execution of your representatives.

Dynamic Appreciation

Dynamic Appreciation is a basic authority device and when utilized really it can fortify the bond among pioneers and workers, guardians and kids and between life partners. Dynamic

Appreciation isn't simply words shared or composed; the study of how our minds functions, neuro-science, demonstrates how the sentiment of gratefulness influences our bodies and conduct of both recipient just as the supplier. Why Active Appreciation rather than just Appreciation? In spite of the fact that, by simply thinking and feeling a feeling of gratefulness can be gainful, it's genuine power is giving it.

Dynamic Is The Key Ingredient

Dynamic conduct is set apart by or including direct investment. It is straightforwardly recognizing or communicating, creating a proposed activity or impact: dynamic fixings. For our talk the dynamic fixing is Appreciation.

Thankfulness is an outflow of appreciation. Dynamic Appreciation is an action word. It implies that pioneers actually give their increase by offering and recognizing their thanks for conduct that supports the associations esteems, mission and business targets.

Reflect for a minute and review a period at work when you felt neglected? How could it feel and what did it do to your inspiration, commitment and responsibility to your exhibition, your chief and the organization? On the off chance that your experience is like mine, those variables diminished and included episodes of self indulgence - which were all non-beneficial for the organization and me.

Pioneers invest a lot of energy seeing what they don't need and typically let representatives realize when they've come up short. Imagine a scenario in which they invested as much energy seeing conduct that supports what they need, and effectively demonstrated their gratefulness for that conduct. Gallup and different investigations demonstrate that we get a greater amount of what we center around. This is the intensity of Active Appreciation; the more you center around effectively acknowledging practices you need, they more your workers will carry on likewise.

Lets accept that your organization esteems

cooperation. What's more, lets expect that a machine needs a support work and that one individual can do it, however on the off chance that someone else helps, it makes the activity simpler, quicker and expands the degree of security. One of your workers consents to play out the upkeep; another administrator makes some noise and says "I have an additional moment, let me help you with it." The subsequent administrator, by offering to help, is exhibiting the soul of cooperation. When you effectively demonstrate your energy about the worker's readiness to help his colleague you are communicating something specific that you esteem cooperation, just as individual execution. By perceiving and effectively acknowledging practices that help and exhibit the qualities you need, you will get a greater amount of it - for this situation, more cooperation, security and thinking about one another.

Stress, Neuro-Science and Active Appreciation

I've heard pioneers allude to worker

commitment and resolve and the abilities that can assemble and fortify these elements as the "delicate stuff". What's more, in monetarily lean and upsetting occasions the "delicate stuff" are commonly the principal things that get cut out. Not exclusively is this reasoning misinformed and awful, the realities don't bolster it. Indeed, the "delicate stuff" and why it works is situated in "hard" science.

I figure we can concur that this violent condition is causing an expansion in worry in pretty much every part of work and family life today. We know from considering individuals that pressure makes changes in the natural chemistry of our bodies and in our conduct. Truth be told, 65% to as high as 85% of the reasons individuals visit their essential consideration doctors is for stress related issues. Stress limits our recognition, decreases intelligent and inventive reasoning and it is related with various physical and intense subject matters. At the point when an individual feels focused on, the cerebrum goes on ready status - prepared to distinguish any apparent danger of peril. It assembles our body to reaction to any apparent risk by discharging a course of hormones, one of which is called cortisol into our circulatory system. Cortisol is proposed to keep the alarm switch on, regardless of whether the apparent danger has passed. Being continually on ready makes us tense and occupied from the work we should be centered around. In the event that you where stranded in a wilderness, your survival would rely upon our being hyper-mindful of the considerable number of risks hiding, and cortisol would be useful. Anyway in an "ordinary" world it neutralizes our capacity to productively and successfully perform. We realize that in the present upsetting workplace that our work isn't typical. It is loaded up with potential dangers and dangers, which are elevated in this recessionary atmosphere. I've had high performing pioneers disclose to me that they have turned out to be agitated and focused on simply catching wind of lay-offs notwithstanding when they've been informed that they don't need to stress. The measure of cortisol streaming in the total circulatory system of the present workforce is running path better than average! This isn't sound for the individual or the hierarchical, which is depending on the exhibition of a couple to keep it focused and gainful.

Neuro-Scientist found another hormone, which has a quieting impact and diminishes the hormones related with pressure, especially cortisol. They found that sentiments of thankfulness and appreciation invigorate the generation of a hormone called oxytocin. The sentiment of being acknowledged produces oxytocin, which kills and diminishes the creation of cortisol, in this way decreasing our useless hyper-carefulness. What's more, there is a connection among ocytocin and the feeling of trust. Furthermore, trust is a fundamental factor in worker duty, steadfastness and execution. At the point when a pioneer centers around and sends gratefulness their like a specialist giving a drug that diminishes pressure and manufactures trust.- helping the worker reestablish and assemble their degree of execution.

Studies have demonstrated that it takes at least 3 positive musings as well as emotions to balance one negative idea or feeling. Concentrates likewise demonstrate that individuals perform better in a situation that is more positive than negative. As referenced, the fierce unpleasant condition that we are encountering makes an adequate inventory of negative contemplations and sentiments. As a pioneer you can help decrease pressure and make a work atmosphere that is progressively gainful by utilizing Active Appreciation to counterbalance the impacts of pressure and the adverse musings and emotions that influence individuals consistently.

CHAPTER SEVEN

Pro-post visit patient calls

For your medicinal practice, the season is at its pinnacle and you are good to go to handle the surge of patients' arrangements feeling that all would be overseen easily. In any case, on the off chance that you think human restorative staff at your social insurance focus is fit enough to take any number of difficulties that may come during everyday administration in pinnacle season, most likely you have left numerous things to consider!

On the off chance that you are a bustling specialist and need to end up quiet as an amphibian in the sun, just hand over the whole medicinal office the executives to Answering Service. Therapeutic Answering System has ability to answers any number of calls from the patients at some random time! Regardless of one patient calling or many! This is helpful component during the restorative camp or inoculation camp, which is free. Besides, the framework accompanies remarkable component of multi-language. You can set the administration in various dialects, for example, Spanish, French, Chinese and English (default). Is it accurate to say that it isn't the most ideal way you can ever need to speak with outsiders as patients?

Other valuable highlights of Answering Service incorporate Patient Reminder System. Utilizing this component, programming can consequently call patients and remind them their inevitable medicinal visits in any capacity whatsoever, for example, body tests, dietary, therapeutic or routine development.

Additionally your patients can be continually reminded about their routine as proposed by you.

One of the most significant zones in restorative office the board is reserving patients arrangements with no blunders. Human restorative assistant, shockingly, is inclined to commit errors and after that covers of time become self-evident. There's another issue every step of the way when time distribution is blundered. To beat this, Nurse Answering Service can fill in as medicinal virtual secretary. It enables the patients to book their arrangements utilizing Internet with no help of medicinal staff at front work area. As such, patients can book their arrangements to see you from anyplace and whenever! Then again, arrangement booking framework can send the information on your iPhone or Smartphone where you can get to the arrangement calendar utilizing Google Synchronization, the remarkable element that the framework has.

During the 1960s, you could call a specialist

to your home with a telephone call. The pattern changed with time. It wound up hard for specialists to head out for long separation to visit patients. With development in medicinal administrations, increasingly restorative professionals worked in gathering practices and therapeutic consideration. With time, the weight on the US human services framework is expanding with patients thinking that its hard to visit emergency clinics and doctors workplaces. Therefore, the quantity of doctors turning towards house calls is additionally expanding. The treatment today is progressively about nurse clinic remain. Crisis cases, patients turn towards clinics for solid consideration.

Patients likewise go to crisis rooms, close by centers in the event that doctors are not accessible for house calls. Individuals get individualized consideration in emergency clinics. With expanding nurse clinic visits, individuals started to approach attendant specialists to spare time on treatment, and to keep away from emergency clinic remain. Patients are additionally redirected to walking facilities for expanded patient volume to clinics.

The pattern of calling specialists to come homes is presently resuscitating again with more doctors picking to move toward becoming house call specialists. The repayment gotten by house call specialists is likewise expanding. The pattern of doctors/specialists at home is back on the grounds that house is the place the patient consideration is required. After 1960s, doctors were making less house calls to patients as a result of weights identified with time and cash. Home visits help specialists in diagnosing and treating wellbeing conditions. The human services expenses are expanding in the US, and patients are moving towards attendant drug to manage it. The normal life expectancy of Americans is longer, and older need to pay more for medicinal services. The pattern is relied upon to proceed for a long time. House call projects require a structure for it to chip away at an enormous scale, for them to work for doctors and patients. A gauge says 4000 doctors made in excess of 2,000,000 out of 2010.

When we headed into this subsidence I think we as a whole realized that we would confront some fascinating issues with our patients when it came to out-of-pocket circumstances. We as a whole can identify with the dread factor of the monetary occasions we are in, for a few of us it is more genuine than others, yet none the less it is genuine. Every day we are seeing indications of it from patients counterbalancing their nurse procedures once they discover they should pay a part, to inquiring as to whether they can post-date checks for copayments.

We comprehend that patients need an incentive from their encounter with the doctor, however as of late we have had more patients call needing "telephone visits" with the specialist so they don't need to pay their copayment or deductible. A considerable lot of these patients need ensures that they will get a treatment at their visit (in the event that they come in) that will fix their concern or they would prefer not to come in. We really had a patient who had not been seen for more than four years call the workplace and inquire as to whether she could drop off x-beams taken by another specialist who would do nurse procedure on her and she need our primary care physician to take a gander at the x-beams and advise her if the system that this specialist needed to perform was right for her. She didn't need an arrangement, only a telephone call would do. It was mind boggling that she figured the specialist would do this.

One patient who was seen for plantar fasciitis was prescribed that she utilize a night support and was indicated what one was. She was determined what her advantages were for this and due to a deductible she said that she would think about it. At her following visit I asked her how she was doing she answered "much better" and I asked what she felt had helped her to improve her indications. She answered "I made a night support out of a cardboard box". Without avoiding a beat I said "bravo, and this is working, which is superb." She was exceptionally upbeat that I was satisfied for her and after that clarified how she made it. I revealed to her she was extremely clever and she said she should have been on the grounds that she had an enormous deductible for sturdy therapeutic gear and since the specialist accepted this gadget would help her she made one. It is astounding what we will do when we are looked with monetary circumstances.

The central matter that I need get crosswise over is the means by which the patient was taken care of. Money related issues are close to home and extreme. Nobody ought to be made to feel that they are considered less in light of the fact that they can't, or don't have any desire to burn through cash out-of-pocket. The inquiry we ought to present ourselves is "how would we hold our patients however extreme occasions?" We have to recall that patients make a statement (they can leave our workplaces for good simply as they strolled in). Covering (Troubled Asset Relief Program, you can Google it) did a social insurance study that indicated the significance of individual treatment in holding patients.

As we have all heard before patients that have negative encounters in our workplaces will discuss these multiple times more than they will discuss the positive ones. This implies you have to make a positive encounter for four patients out of each five you see. At the point when issues raise patients are bound to bring negligence activities against a doctor on the off chance that they are not happy with how they have been dealt with. At the point when patients are happy with their treatment at the workplace they are bound to be progressively agreeable with treatment systems, so they will create better results.

We have to raise our affectability mindfulness level when chatting with our patients about treatment that would resolve their concern, yet are revealed by their protection. In our office we used to call patients with their advantages for tough medicinal hardware, PT, nurse procedure, and so forth., to tell them their inclusion and found that multiple occasions in the event that they didn't have inclusion or had a deductible they would not plan an arrangement to return, they would disclose to us they would consider it and get back to, yet never did. These patients felt that if the treatment the specialist needed them to have was revealed or distant monetarily for them, at that point why returned? We have since changed how we handle this and reappoint the patient while they are in the workplace and told them that we will check their advantages and talk about them at that arrangement. At that point in the event that they don't have inclusion or have a deductible we can talk about this vis-à-vis with them, which is a more close to home method for correspondence than via telephone. We are setting aside the effort to identify with our patients by talking and tuning in to them. In the event that it isn't something the patient can do as of now, that is alright, the specialist would then be able to alter the treatment plan likewise with the patient regardless they get care. It is a success win for all.

At the point when our patients are glad the specialists and staff are upbeat and our office condition is lovely, which decreases burnout, stress and disappointment in our employments. We have to take a stab at magnificence in our workplaces offering an incentive to our patients as close to home connections. Issues and difficulties will consistently come up, yet the manner in which we handle them that will have the effect. These difficulties are openings that are basic to our prosperity with our patients and our training.

CONCLUSION

Being a diligent nurse attendant is altogether different from different claims to fame, in light of the fact that careful nurse attendants manage patients who are sleeping. Careful attendants see the patients quickly in pre-operation and afterward return them to the working room where they will be put to rest by either an Anesthesiologist or a Certified Registered Nurse Anesthetist (CRNA).

Careful nurse caretakers are extremely regional and strange. Nobody else truly realizes what goes on behind those OR entryways, (neither patients or different nurse caretakers). It's a totally extraordinary world in nurse procedure and without the best possible preparing, you're not allowed to enter the careful zone.

Careful attendants don't change dressings; they more often than not don't direct meds (with the exception of neighborhood checking). They don't answer call lights or manage patients' families. So what the hell do they do?

All things considered, behind those careful entryways are some astoundingly prepared nurse attendants who merit acknowledgment and commendation, which is something they once in a while get.

They don't perceive how a patient recoup. The patients are so high on Versed that they have amnesia after their entire careful experience.

www.ingramcontent.com/pod-product-compliance
Lightning Source LLC
Chambersburg PA
CBHW070539220526
45467CB00003B/993